T0263488

The Hallux

Guest Editor

JOHN T. CAMPBELL, MD

FOOT AND ANKLE CLINICS

www.foot.theclinics.com

Consulting Editor
MARK S. MYERSON, MD

March 2009 • Volume 14 • Number 1

SAUNDERS an imprint of ELSEVIER, Inc.

W.B. SAUNDERS COMPANY
A Division of Elsevier Inc.

1600 John F. Kennedy Blvd. ● Suite 1800 ● Philadelphia, PA 19103-2899

http://www.theclinics.com

FOOT AND ANKLE CLINICS Volume 14, Number 1
March 2009 ISSN 1083-7515, ISBN-10: 1-4377-0475-1, ISBN-13: 978-1-4377-0475-4

Editor: Debora Dellapena

Foot and Ankle Clinics (ISSN 1083-7515) is published quarterly by Elsevier, Inc., 360 Park Avenue South, New York, NY 10010-1710. Months of issue are March, June, September, and December. Business and Editorial Offices: 1600 John F. Kennedy Blvd., Suite 1800, Philadelphia, PA 19103-2899. Customer Service Office: 11830 Westline Industrial Drive, St. Louis, MO 63146. Periodicals postage paid at New York, NY, and additional mailing offices. Subscription price per year is $230.00 (US individuals), $333.00 (US institutions), $116.00 (US students), $257.00 (Canadian individuals), $394.00 (Canadian institutions), $159.00 (Canadian students), $331.00 (foreign individuals), $394.00 (foreign institutions), and $159.00 (foreign students). To receive student/resident rate, orders must be accompanied by name of affiliated institution, date of term, and the *signature* of program/residency coordinator on institution letterhead. Orders will be billed at individual rate until proof of status is received. Foreign air speed delivery is included in all *Clinics* subscription prices. All prices are subject to change without notice. **POSTMASTER:** Send address changes to *Foot and Ankle Clinics*, Elsevier Periodicals Customer Service, 11830 Westline Industrial Drive, St. Louis, MO 63146. **Customer Service: 1-800-654-2452 (US). From outside of the United States, call 314-453-7041. Fax: 314-453-5170. E-mail: JournalsCustomerService-usa@elsevier.com (for print support); JournalsOnlineSupport-usa@elsevier. com (for online support).**

Reprints. For copies of 100 or more, of articles in this publication, please contact the Commercial Reprints Department, Elsevier Inc., 360 Park Avenue South, New York, NY 10010-1710. Tel.: 212-633-3812; Fax: 212-462-1935; E-mail: reprints@elsevier.com.

Printed and bound in the United Kingdom
Transferred to Digital Print 2011

Contributors

CONSULTING EDITOR

MARK S. MYERSON, MD
Director, Institute for Foot and Ankle Reconstruction at Mercy, Mercy Medical Center, Baltimore, Maryland

GUEST EDITOR

JOHN T. CAMPBELL, MD
Institute for Foot and Ankle Reconstruction at Mercy, Mercy Medical Center, Baltimore, Maryland

AUTHORS

ADAM BECKER, MD
Englewood Orthopedic Associates, Englewood, New Jersey

DOMINIC S. CARREIRA, MD
Broward Health Orthopedics, Fort Lauderdale, Florida

BRUCE E. COHEN, MD
Fellowship Director, OrthoCarolina Foot and Ankle Institute, Charlotte, North Carolina

BERNHARD DEVOS BEVERNAGE, MD
Orthopaedic Surgeon, Department of Orthopaedic Surgery, Saint-Luc University Hospital, Brussels, Belgium

SUSAN N. ISHIKAWA, MD
Associate Professor, Fellowship Director, University of Tennessee, Campbell Clinic, Collierville, Tennessee

ANISH R. KADAKIA, MD
Chief, Division of Foot and Ankle Surgery, Department of Orthopedic Surgery; and Instructor, Department of Orthopaedic Surgery, University of Michigan Hospitals, Ann Arbor, Michigan

THIBAUT LEEMRIJSE, MD
Orthopaedic Surgeon, Professor, Department of Orthopaedic Surgery, Saint-Luc University Hospital, Brussels, Belgium

RICHARD M. MARKS, MD, FACS
Professor, Department of Orthopaedic Surgery, Director, Division of Foot and Ankle Surgery, Medical College of Wisconsin, Milwaukee, Wisconsin

STUART D. MILLER, MD
Department of Orthopaedic Surgery, Union Memorial Hospital, Baltimore, Maryland

NICHOLAS R. SEIBERT, MD
Chief Resident, Department of Orthopaedic Surgery, University of Michigan Hospitals, Ann Arbor, Michigan

PAUL S. SHURNAS, MD
Director, Orthopaedic Foot and Ankle Surgery, Columbia Orthopaedic Group, Columbia, Missouri

MARTIN R. SULLIVAN, MBBS (Hon), FRACS, FAOrthA
Foot and Ankle Surgeon, St. Vincent's Clinic, Sydney, Australia

JOHN W. WOMACK, MD
Clinical Instructor, Piedmont Orthopaedic Associates, Greenville, South Carolina

Contents

> Hallux rigidus is a degenerative osteoarthritic process characterized by progressive loss of metatarsophalangeal joint range of motion and notable dorsal or periarticular osteophyte formation. Documented factors associated with hallux rigidus are a flat or chevron-shaped joint, hallux valgus interphalangeus, metatarsus adductus, bilaterality in persons with a positive family history, trauma history in unilateral cases, and female gender. Elevation of the first ray noted radiographically is thought to be a sign of worsening metatarsophalangeal joint function. Nonoperative care is aimed at improving comfort of the toe and foot with roomy shoes, selective joint injections, taping, and selective use of orthotics.

> Cheilectomy has long been the standard treatment in the orthopedic community for mild to moderate cases of hallux rigidus, with established long-term excellent results. Osteotomies of the proximal phalanx and first metatarsal have been described mainly in the podiatric literature; they have shown good outcomes in small patient groups with short-term follow-up. Proper patient selection is critical to obtaining favorable outcomes with any of the joint-sparing procedures. Patients with severe arthritic changes and pain in the midrange arc of motion have poorer outcomes with these procedures and are better served with joint-destructive procedures, such as arthroplasty or arthrodesis.

> The treatment of advanced hallux rigidus in an older, more sedentary population with poor bone stock or comorbidities that may make corrective osteotomy, fusion, and implant fixation more problematic has frequently been an issue for orthopedic surgeons. The traditional Keller resection

arthroplasty has not fared well because of various problems. Crescentic oblique basilar resection arthroplasty is a viable surgical treatment alternative for older, more sedentary patients who have advanced hallux rigidus with or without hallux valgus. This may also be a good alternative procedure in a more active patient who wishes to avoid fusion of the joint while maintaining some first MTP motion.

Hallux rigidus or osteoarthritis of the first metatarsophalangeal joint is characterized by pain, stiffness of the joint, and alterations of gait. The appeal of joint arthroplasty for hallux rigidus is similar to its benefits in other joints in the body. The ideal implant should relieve pain, restore motion, improve function, and maintain joint stability. Numerous implants have been described for the hallux metatarsophalangeal joint. This article discusses various implant options along with clinical outcomes and complications.

Arthrodesis of the first metatarsophalangeal joint is a highly successful treatment for patients with symptomatic hallux rigidus who have failed conservative management. Before arthrodesis, the importance of host factors, such as use of nicotine, local blood supply, medical comorbidites, and use of systemic immunosuppressive agents, must be considered. Arthrodesis is currently considered the gold standard treatment for end-stage arthritis of the metatarsophalangeal joint. Careful attention to surgical detail is critical to achieving optimal outcomes.

Appropriate treatment for hallux varus requires comprehensive radiographic and systematic clinical assessment to identify the involved factors. A classification scheme must incorporate many variables in order to determine the best approach to correcting the deformity. This article focuses on iatrogenic hallux varus following bunion surgery, but the same principles apply to other causes of acquired hallux varus.

Nerve disorders about the hallux can generate remarkable pain and dysfunction. Whether caused by soft tissue entrapment, trauma, iatrogenic injury, or from an idiopathic basis; nerve disorders are approached by careful history and examination followed by nonoperative treatment. In cases that do not respond, meticulous surgical management can be helpful in many cases.

Malunion of a first metatarsal osteotomy or fracture can result in dorsal angulation of the distal fragment and shortening of the metatarsal, among other deformities. Dorsal malunion can be caused by improper orientation of the osteotomy, poor intraoperative fixation, or loss of fixation post-operatively due to premature weight bearing or catastrophic failure. There is little in the literature on the rate and incidence of malunion following first metatarsal fractures treated either operatively or nonoperatively. However, treatment options would be similar as for malunion following an osteotomy. The treatment of malunions depends on how symptomatic the patient is, including pain, difficulty with ambulation, and whether they complain of transfer metatarsalgia.

Sesamoid disorders are common causes of forefoot pain. Because of the significant mechanical stresses and anatomic variations involved, the sesamoid complex appears to be affected by numerous pathologic processes. These include acute fractures, stress fractures, nonunions, osteonecrosis, chondromalacia, and various inflammatory conditions labeled sesamoiditis. Treatment options include conservative management with orthotics and immobilization, as well as operative interventions that range from fracture/nonunion fixation to various approaches for sesamoidectomy. This article outlines the diagnosis and treatment of these entities and reviews the results of these treatments.

Arthroscopy of the first MTP joint is a useful, minimally invasive technique in treating a number of pathologies about the hallux MTP joint. However, it is a technically demanding procedure for which there is a learning curve. The small arthroscope and instrumentation are delicate and vulnerable to damage. Practice on cadavers is very useful in shortening this learning curve, and experience with arthroscopy in other joints facilitates the transition to the hallux. In the future, additional studies will help to more specifically define the indications and expected outcomes of treatment as such will help to further elucidate the potential benefits over open surgery.

THE CLINICS ARE NOW AVAILABLE ONLINE!

Access your subscription at:
www.theclinics.com

Foreword

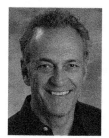

Mark S. Myerson, MD
Consulting Editor

Surgical correction of hallux rigidus is fairly predictable, and patient acceptance and outcome should be good. There are many surgical alternatives to choose from, all based on the underlying anatomy, the pathology, and the extent of arthritis. To some extent, patient needs for activities and shoe wear do play a role, but in general, this should not influence the decision making for the type of surgery.

By and large the surgical management of hallux rigidus has not changed very much over the past few decades, and this is a good observation, since it implies that what we are doing works. Certainly, in my own practice a cheilectomy, with or without an osteotomy at the base of the proximal phalanx, is the most predictable operation for correction of hallux rigidus. Perhaps the most significant finding regarding the use of cheilectomy is when it is used for more advanced forms of arthritis. From a functional and biological standpoint, there is no reason why a cheilectomy for severe impingement and arthritis should work, and yet unpredictably, it does. I have observed that many patients return years following a cheilectomy for further treatment, but on the opposite foot. When obtaining an Xray, it may seem that the operated foot appears far worse than the now symptomatic foot. Why is this? Is there perhaps some denervation of the joint which takes place during cheilectomy? Is the mechanical decompression sufficient for management of most patients? One would presume that the latter would be correct, since the kinematics of the joint are never normalized following cheilectomy, regardless of the severity of the disease process. For management of the more severe grades of arthritis, although I perform arthrodesis frequently, I have experienced excellent results from interposition arthroplasty, yet despite efforts with various implants, have experienced less than desirable results with various types of implant arthroplasty.

Arthrodesis continues to be a mainstay of treatment in the management of severe arthritis associated with deformity or when other salvage procedures in the forefoot need to be performed simultaneously. Occasionally, osteotomy of the first metatarsal is advantageous. Elevation of the first metatarsal may not have a significant role in the pathogenesis of hallux rigidus, but there is a most definite correlation between metatarsus elevatus and more severe grades of hallux rigidus. Furthermore, a distal oblique metatarsal osteotomy in the manner of a triple osteotomy used to correct the lesser

Foot Ankle Clin N Am 14 (2009) ix–x
doi:10.1016/j.fcl.2008.12.002
1083-7515/08/$ – see front matter © 2009 Elsevier Inc. All rights reserved.

metatarsal deformity (after Maceira), is very useful for the patient who has a long and elevated 1st metatarsal. Osteotomy of the metatarsal or arthrodesis of the 1st tarsometatarsal joint must also be part of a surgical treatment armamentarium in which the 1st metatarsal is markedly elevated and unstable. This is particularly the case when the joint appears to be normal, and the metatarsal is long and elevated, probably indicating that jamming of the joint occurs in push off. Lastly, there is a group of patients who do not "fit" the typical diagnosis of hallux rigidus, since they have good range of motion, but joint pain due to early arthritis. Intraoperative findings usually indicate a central osteochondral defect of the metatarsal head, which requires treatment. An osteochondral graft can be harvested from the normal dorsal aspect of the joint, a free osteochondral autograft used, or a synthetic bi-phasic graft. The results of treatment are generally good, however things go wrong when the expectations of the patient are not met, not necessarily when biology and mechanics fail.

Mark S. Myerson, MD
Director
Institute for Foot and Ankle Reconstruction at Mercy
Mercy Medical Center
301 St. Paul Place
Baltimore, MD 21202, USA

E-mail address:
Mark4feet@aol.com

Preface

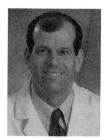

John T. Campbell, MD
Guest Editor

The hallux and first ray play a crucial role in stance, ambulation, and propulsion. During stance phase, normal gait demonstrates progression of pressure through the foot, terminating in the hallux. Disorders of the hallux and first metatarsal can impair this function, resulting in dramatic effects on gait. Hallux valgus has commanded significant attention as a disorder that alters forefoot mechanics and disrupts patients' function. Other conditions of the hallux and first ray may draw less attention, but can similarly cause severe pain and impairment. This issue of *Foot and Ankle Clinics* will focus on these other topics, some of which are common and others which are esoteric but no less important.

A series of authors have focused in depth on hallux rigidus. The etiology and pathophysiology of this condition are covered, followed by proper evaluation and nonoperative treatments. Surgical options are then explored in depth, covering cheilectomy, metatarsal and phalangeal osteotomies, resection and interposition arthroplasties, implant arthroplasty, and arthrodesis. The authors are to be commended for exploring in detail the proper indications, meticulous operative techniques, postoperative management, and outcomes of these varied approaches.

Other articles address iatrogenic problems, including malunion, nonunion and osteonecrosis of the first metatarsal, nerve disorders of the hallux, and the challenging problem of hallux varus deformity. These authors lead the reader through etiology, clinical evaluation, and treatment options to properly manage these troublesome conditions. Sesamoid disorders occur due to numerous etiologies, affecting athletes and non-athletes alike. A discussion of causative factors along with a methodical approach to diagnosis and management is presented. Arthroscopy of the first metatarsophalangeal joint has improved with advances in small joint arthroscopic equipment and instrumentation; a comprehensive guide is provided, including proper indications, patient set-up, and surgical techniques.

Foot Ankle Clin N Am 14 (2009) xi–xii
doi:10.1016/j.fcl.2008.12.001
1083-7515/08/$ – see front matter © 2009 Elsevier Inc. All rights reserved.

foot.theclinics.com

A diverse panel of experts has been assembled to provide experienced insight into the appropriate management of these challenging problems, whether common or unusual. We hope that our efforts will assist in the treatment of patients, leading ultimately to improved function and quality of life.

John T. Campbell, MD
Institute for Foot and Ankle Reconstruction at Mercy
Mercy Medical Center
301 St. Paul Place
Baltimore, MD 21202, USA

E-mail address:
jcampbell@mdmercy.com

Hallux Rigidus: Etiology, Biomechanics, and Nonoperative Treatment

Paul S. Shurnas, MD

KEYWORDS

- Osteoarthritis • Rigidus • Hallux • Limitus
- Inherited • Bilateral

ETIOLOGY AND BIOMECHANICS

The term "hallux rigidus" describes a painful malady of the great toe metatarsophalangeal (MTP) joint characterized primarily by loss of dorsiflexion and progressive osteophyte formation about the MTP joint. Initially the condition was reported in 1887 by Davies-Colley,[1] who described a plantar-flexed position of the proximal phalanx relative to the metatarsal head and proposed "hallux flexus." Cotterill[2] reported on the same condition a few months later, however, and suggested the diagnosis of hallux rigidus. The commonly used terms "hallux rigidus" and "hallux limitus" are used to describe degrees of the same problem. DuVries[3] and Moberg[4] noted that other than hallux valgus, hallux rigidus is the most common problem of the first MTP joint.

The literature shows a higher incidence of female involvement.[5–10] Coughlin[7] reported that approximately 80% of patients with bilateral hallux rigidus had a history in their family of great toe arthritis or "bunions." Long-term follow-up of the same patients with hallux rigidus showed that more than 80% developed bilateral disease. Although numerous contributory factors have been hypothesized, there has been no proven association or correlation with first ray mobility, metatarsal length, Achilles or gastrocnemius contracture, planovalgus or cavus foot posture, hallux valgus, adolescent onset, type of shoe wear, occupation, or metatarsus primus elevatus.[7,11]

Trauma is the most common cause reported in the literature and may occur as a single, isolated injury (eg, fracture) or possibly the result of chronic repetitive microtrauma.[12] A traumatic episode is the most likely cause of unilateral hallux rigidus.[7] An injury that results in forced hyperextension[12] or plantar flexion (PF)[13]

Orthopaedic Foot and Ankle Surgery, Columbia Orthopaedic Group, 1 South Keene Street, Columbia, MO 65201, USA
E-mail address: pjshurnas@juno.com

Foot Ankle Clin N Am 14 (2009) 1–8
doi:10.1016/j.fcl.2008.11.001

may create compressive and shear forces that result in chondral or osteochondral injury. The resultant joint damage leads to progressive arthritic changes over time. A severe sprain or "turf toe" injury also may develop into arthritis. Younger, active patients with hallux rigidus may present after a sprain or jamming episode with an osteochondral defect of the MTP joint, but the diagnosis can be difficult, and oblique radiographs and MRI may be helpful.[14–18]

Other factors associated with hallux rigidus in the literature include a flat or chevron-shaped joint, metatarsus adductus, hallux valgus interphalangeus, bilaterality in persons with a positive family history, trauma in unilateral cases, and female gender.[6,7,19] The notion that instability of the first ray may predispose to hallux valgus is the corollary to the notion that a flat or chevron-shaped joint can lead to hallux rigidus. Such a constrained joint (congenital or acquired) may result more easily in jamming episodes and the resultant degenerative changes. Metatarsus adductus may be another underlying factor that creates abnormal stress on the MTP joint, but more research is needed regarding these potential causes to determine the mechanism.

Metatarsus primus elevatus (**Fig. 1**) is classically described as a fixed dorsal elevation of the first metatarsal in relation to the lesser metatarsals. For example, fixed elevation may occur iatrogenically after a first metatarsal osteotomy or may be caused by fracture malunion. Flexible elevation has been associated with posterior tibial

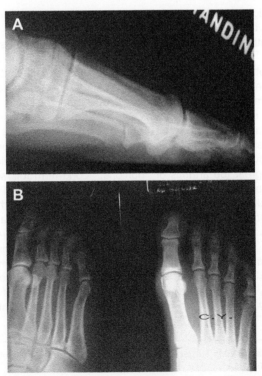

Fig. 1. Grade 1 hallux rigidus. (*A*) The lateral radiograph shows elevation of the first ray (elevatus) and often is the key finding in early grades to suggest hallux rigidus. (*B*) The metatarsal head is enlarged and the dorsal surface is prominent. Loose bodies and sesamoid irregularity are not obvious but may occur with any grade.

tendon deficiency, peroneal weakness, spastic conditions, and even paralysis. Recent studies evaluated metatarsus primus elevatus in patients with hallux rigidus.[7,11,19] Based on these studies, metatarsus primus elevatus was a secondary condition that correlated well with arthritic progression, severity of arthritis, and loss of MTP joint range of motion. Metatarsus primus elevatus was nearly eliminated after hallux rigidus repair, interposition arthroplasty, and arthrodesis. Meyer and colleagues[20] found no statistical correlation between hallux rigidus and first metatarsal elevation. They reported that up to 5 mm of elevation was considered normal. Horton and Myerson[21] confirmed Meyer's study and documented no association with hallux rigidus. The author believes that metatarsus primus elevatus is more useful as a diagnostic aid to help diagnose early or subtle cases of hallux rigidus and has noted decreased elevation after selective MTP joint injections and improvement of first ray weight bearing on dynamic gait studies. More profound first ray elevation is usually noted with advancing hallux rigidus.

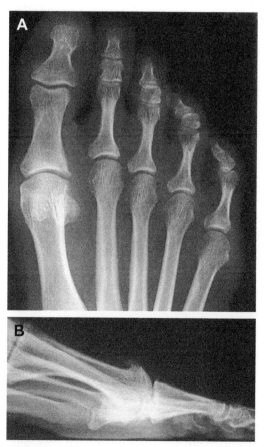

Fig. 2. Grade 2 hallux rigidus. (*A*) The metatarsal head is more flattened, marginal osteophytes are notable, and increased elevatus is obvious on the lateral radiograph. (*B*) The dorsal osteophyte is often the key finding on the lateral radiograph and classically appears like dripping candle wax. The joint space is fairly well preserved, but increased subchondral radiodensity is noted.

Clinical Findings

Early hallux rigidus is characterized by synovial thickening, MTP joint inflammation, and mild restriction in MTP joint motion. Patients may have flares of swelling and pain, but over time the flare-ups become more frequent, the joint begins to enlarge, and symptoms become more pronounced. Wearing shoes becomes difficult and most patients seek medical attention out of concern that they may have gout or a broken toe. The primary pathologic process of hallux rigidus is degenerative arthritis.[16] The common location of cartilage depletion is on the dorsal portion of the metatarsal head.[4,22] As the degeneration progresses, dorsal and dorsolateral osteophytes on the metatarsal head become pronounced and the bony ridge may impinge against the proximal phalanx (**Figs. 2–4**).

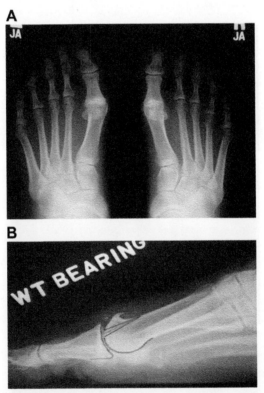

Fig. 3. Grade 3 hallux rigidus. (*A*) The first MTP joint has a definite flat appearance with proliferating marginal osteophytes, loss of cartilage space, and loose body formation. Clinically, patients have a stiff toe (10° of dorsiflexion typically) but no pain at the mid-range of the joint. Primarily they have pain at the extremes of motion caused by impingement of the dorsal osteophyte. The elevatus is markedly increased and the radiodensity around the joint is increased compared with grade 2. Elevatus is associated with worsening MTP joint function. Hallux interphalangeus (angular deformity of the proximal phalanx) is clearly notable and is associated with advanced hallux rigidus—often grades 2, 3, and 4. (*B*) The lateral radiograph demonstrates some plantar cartilage space remaining.

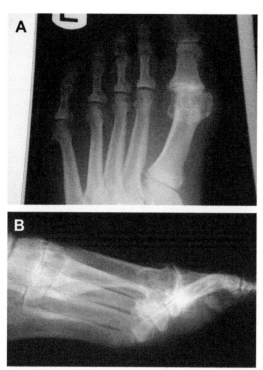

Fig. 4. Grade 4 hallux rigidus. (*A*) Grade 4 changes are often the same as grade 3; the key distinguishing factor is clinical. Grade 4 patients have pain at the mid-range of MTP joint motion with gentle loading, which indicates complete loss of cartilage. (*B*) Radiographs usually demonstrate complete cartilage space loss, especially on the lateral view.

Physical examination demonstrates a tender, painful, swollen MTP joint that exhibits limited motion. Grinding, catching, or clicking may be present, and with joint motion, pain may be elicited in dorsiflexion, plantarflexion, or both. Pain that clearly occurs at the mid-range of motion with gentle loading indicates profound MTP joint cartilage loss. Osteophyte growth around the margin of the affected joint may cause a superficial bursitis, neuritis, or skin ulceration. Interphalangeal joint hyperextension may be noted as compensation for restricted MTP joint dorsiflexion.[23,24]

Radiographic findings

Radiographs usually show asymmetric loss of cartilage space or chondrolysis, subchondral cysts evident in advancing cases, increased sclerosis and bony proliferation at the joint margins, and loose bodies around the joint. Standing anteroposterior, oblique, and lateral radiographs of the foot are sufficient in most cases. The anteroposterior view often shows the asymmetric joint narrowing and a flattened widening of the metatarsal head. In more advanced stages, cystic changes in the metatarsal, increased radiodensity, osteophyte formation on the base of the proximal phalanx, and sesamoid enlargement usually develop. The lateral radiograph may demonstrate a dorsal metatarsal osteophyte classic for "dripping candle wax" as the osteophyte courses proximally along the dorsal metatarsal surface. A radiographic and clinical classification system helps to define the magnitude of the arthritic process and may help select specific nonoperative or operative treatment (**Box 1**).[19]

Box 1

Clinical and radiographic classification of hallux rigidus

Grade 0

    ROM: Dorsiflexion 40°–60° and/or 10%–20% loss compared with normal side

    Radiograph: normal or minimal findings

    Clinical: no subjective pain, only stiffness, loss of passive motion on examination

Grade 1

    ROM: Dorsiflexion 30°–40° and/or 20%–50% loss compared with normal side

    Radiograph: dorsal spur is main finding, minimal joint narrowing, minimal periarticular sclerosis, minimal flattening of metatarsal head

    Clinical: mild or occasional subjective pain and stiffness, pain at extremes of dorsiflexion and/or plantarflexion on examination

Grade 2

    ROM: Dorsiflexion 10°–30° and/or 50%–75% loss compared with normal side

    Radiograph: dorsal, lateral and possibly medial osteophytes give flattened appearance to metatarsal head, no more than one fourth of dorsal joint space involvement on lateral radiograph, mild to moderate joint narrowing and sclerosis, sesamoids not usually involved but may be irregular in appearance

    Clinical: moderate to severe subjective pain and stiffness that may be constant, pain just before maximal dorsiflexion and/or plantarflexion on examination

Grade 3

    ROM: Dorsiflexion of 10° or less and/or 75%–100% loss compared with normal side and notable loss of plantarflexion (often ≤ 10° PF).

    Radiograph: as in Grade 2 but with substantial narrowing, possibly periarticular cystic changes, more than one fourth dorsal joint may be involved on lateral, sesmoids (enlarged and/or cystic and/or irregular)

    Clinical: nearly constant subjective pain and substantial stiffness, pain throughout ROM on examination (but not at mid-range)

Grade 4

    Same criteria and findings as Grade 3, but definite pain at mid-ROM on examination is elicited

Abbreviation: ROM, Range of motion.
Data from Coughlin MJ, Shurnas PS. Hallux rigidus: grading and long-term results of operative treatment. J Bone Joint Surg Am 2003;85A:2072–88.

NONSURGICAL TREATMENT

Nonoperative treatment of symptomatic hallux rigidus must be tailored to each patient depending on the extent of arthritis and symptoms. The proper diagnosis must be obtained and inflammatory conditions be ruled out when necessary with appropriate blood work or joint aspiration. Early disease (grades 0–2) is often treatable with anti-inflammatory medications, shoe stretching, and strapping of the toe with figure of eight tape or Coban wrap. If symptoms continue or worsen, the use of a stiff insole (Morton's extension) to reduce excursion of the MTP joint may be useful. Orthoses have been shown to yield better long-term pain relief than nonsteroidal anti-inflamma-tory drugs alone.[25] The inserts can be moved from shoe to shoe. Unfortunately, with later disease (advanced grade 2 and grades 3–4) some orthotics reduce room in the toe box and may create pressure on the dorsal prominence. Consequently, shoes with a deeper toe box are recommended. Orthotics with a supportive arch decrease pronation, which potentially alleviates pressure on the MTP joint. A carbon-fiber reinforcement under the first ray acts like a Morton's extension to minimize MTP joint excursion.

Solan and colleagues[26] noted 6 months of clinical improvement with intra-articular steroid injection and gentle MTP joint manipulation for mild to moderate grades of hallux rigidus. The same authors found limited benefit in more advanced grades, however. Smith and colleagues[27] reported on the long-term follow-up of 22 patients (24 feet) treated nonsurgically for hallux rigidus with a mean follow-up of 14 years. The authors reported that 75% of patients continued to choose nonoperative treatment, although the intensity of pain remained the same in 22 feet, worsened in 1 foot, and improved in 1 foot. Most patients were able to tolerate their pain by wearing a roomy, stiff-soled shoe. Others reported 60% successful nonoperative results with 1 to 7 years of follow-up using shoe wear modifications, orthoses, injections, and taping.[28]

REFERENCES

1. Davies-Colley M. Contraction of the metatarsophalangeal joint of the great toe. Br Med J 1887;1:728.
2. Cotterill J. Stiffness of the great toe in adolescents. Br Med J 1888;1:1158.
3. DuVries H. Static deformities. In: DuVries H, editor. Surgery of the foot. St. Louis (MO): Mosby; 1959. p. 392–8.
4. Moberg E. A simple operation for hallux rigidus. Clin Orthop Relat Res 1979;142:55–6.
5. Bonney G, Macnab I. Hallux valgus and hallux rigidus: a critical survey of opera-tive results. J Bone Joint Surg Br 1952;34B:366–85.
6. Coughlin MJ, Mann RA. Arthrodesis of the first metatarsophalangeal joint as salvage for the failed Keller procedure. J Bone Joint Surg Am 1987;69A:68–75.
7. Coughlin MJ, Shurnas PS. Hallux rigidus: demographics, etiology, and radiographic assessment. Foot Ankle Int 2003;24:731–43.
8. Drago JJ, Oloff L, Jacobs AM, et al. A comprehensive review of hallux limitus. J Foot Surg 1984;23:213–20.
9. Mann RA, Clanton TO. Hallux rigidus: treatment by cheilectomy. J Bone Joint Surg Am 1988;70A:400–6.
10. Nilsonne H. Hallux rigidus and its treatment. Acta Orthop Scand 1930;1:295–303.
11. Coughlin MJ, Shurnas PS. Soft-tissue arthroplasty for hallux rigidus. Foot Ankle Int 2003;24:661–72.
12. Coughlin MJ. Conditions of the forefoot. In: DeLee J, Drez D, editors. Ortho-paedic sports medicine: principles and practice. Philadelphia: WB Saunders; 1994. p. 221–44.
13. Frey C, Andersen GD, Feder KS, et al. Plantarflexion injury to the metatarsopha-langeal joint ("sand toe"). Foot Ankle Int 1996;17:576–81.
14. Goodfellow J. Aetiology of hallux rigidus. Proc R Soc Med 1966;59:821–4.
15. Hanft JR, Mason ET, Landsman AS, et al. A new radiographic classification for hallux limitus. J Foot Ankle Surg 1993;32:397–404.

16. Kessel L, Bonney G. Hallux rigidus in the adolescent. J Bone Joint Surg Br 1958; 40B:669–73.
17. McMaster MJ. The pathogenesis of hallux rigidus. J Bone Joint Surg Br 1978;60B: 82–7.
18. Schweitzer ME, Maheshwari S, Shabshin N, et al. Hallux valgus and hallux rigidus: MRI findings. Clin Imaging 1999;23:397–402.
19. Coughlin MJ, Shurnas PS. Hallux rigidus: grading and long-term results of operative treatment. J Bone Joint Surg Am 2003;85A:2072–88.
20. Meyer JO, Nishon LR, Weiss L, et al. Metatarsus primus elevatus and the etiology of hallux rigidus. J Foot Surg 1987;26:237–41.
21. Horton GA, Park YW, Myerson MS, et al. Role of metatarsus primus elevatus in the pathogenesis of hallux rigidus. Foot Ankle Int 1999;20:777–80.
22. Hattrup SJ, Johnson KA. Subjective results of hallux rigidus following treatment with cheilectomy. Clin Orthop Relat Res 1988;226:182–91.
23. Feldman RS, Hutter J, Lapow L, et al. Cheilectomy and hallux rigidus. J Foot Surg 1983;22:170–4.
24. Gould N. Hallux rigidus: cheilotomy or implant? Foot Ankle 1981;1:315–20.
25. Thompson JA, Jennings MB, Hodge W, et al. Orthotic therapy in the management of osteoarthritis. J Am Podiatr Med Assoc 1992;82:136–9.
26. Solan MC, Calder JD, Bendall SP, et al. Manipulation and injection for hallux rigidus: is it worthwhile? J Bone Joint Surg Br 2001;83B:706–8.
27. Smith RW, Katchis SD, Ayson LC, et al. Outcomes in hallux rigidus patients treated nonoperatively: a long-term follow-up study. Foot Ankle Int 2000;21: 906–13.
28. Grady JF, Axe TM, Zager EJ, et al. A retrospective analysis of 772 patients with hallux limitus. J Am Podiatr Med Assoc 2002;92:102–8.

Surgical Management of Hallux Rigidus: Cheilectomy and Osteotomy (Phalanx and Metatarsal)

Nicholas R. Seibert, MD[a], Anish R. Kadakia, MD[a,b],*

KEYWORDS

• Hallux rigidus • Cheilectomy • Osteotomy • Phalanx
• Metatarsal • Management

Hallux rigidus is defined as degenerative arthritis of the first metatarsophalangeal (MTP) joint that results in pain and decreased range of motion, primarily dorsiflexion. The pathology was originally described by Davies-Colley in 1887,[1] who termed the disorder hallux flexus. The term "hallux rigidus" was introduced 4 months later by Cotterill,[2] and this description remains the most commonly used name. Multiple causes have been proposed to cause hallux rigidus. Traumatic injury to the articular cartilage has been suggested[3] as a mechanism. A long first metatarsal has been proposed as the cause by Nilsonne[4] and Bonney and Macnab.[5] Lambrinudi[6] introduced the concept of metatarsus primus elevatus, proposing that an elevated first metatarsal leads to plantarflexion of the toe and development of a flexion contracture. The proposed causes of a long first metatarsal and metatarsus primus elevatus are the underlying basis for many of the osteotomies designed to treat this condition.

GRADING

The most common grading system used in the orthopedic literature is that of Hattrup and Johnson.[7] The classification is based on radiographic changes of the first MTP joint on standing anteroposterior and lateral radiographic examination of the foot. Grade I changes consist of mild to moderate osteophyte formation with joint space

[a] Department of Orthopaedic Surgery, University of Michigan Hospitals, 1500 E Medical Center Drive, Taubman Center 2914, Ann Arbor, MI 48109, Michigan, USA
[b] Division of Foot and Ankle Surgery, Department of Orthopaedic Surgery, University of Michigan Hospitals, Division of Foot and Ankle Surgery, 2098 S Main Street, Ann Arbor, MI 48103, Michigan, USA
* Corresponding author.
E-mail address: anishk@med.umich.edu (A.R. Kadakia).

Foot Ankle Clin N Am 14 (2009) 9–22
doi:10.1016/j.fcl.2008.11.002
1083-7515/08/$ – see front matter © 2009 Elsevier Inc. All rights reserved.

preservation. Grade II changes exist if there is less than 50% joint space narrowing, subchondral sclerosis, and moderate osteophyte formation (**Fig. 1**). Grade III changes result when there is marked osteophyte formation and more than 50% loss of visible joint space, with or without subchondral cyst formation. This classification is important when determining treatment, because joint-sparing procedures (see later discussion) are often successful when used for grade I and II diseases. Joint-sparing procedures yield poorer results with grade III disease, which is more appropriately treated by joint ablation procedures, such as resection arthroplasty and arthrodesis.

CHEILECTOMY

Cheilectomy is defined as excision of the dorsal exostosis and the degenerative portion of the articular surface of the first metatarsal head (**Fig. 2**). It was first described by Nilsonne[4] in 1930 when he used the technique in two patients but felt that it only resulted in temporary relief. Bonney and Macnab[5] reviewed their experience from 1920 to 1950, during which 9 of 56 ft with hallux rigidus underwent excision of the exostosis alone. They found poor results and only advocated the procedure for "cases with polyarthritis, or with symptoms referable solely to an exostosis." DuVries[8] popularized the procedure in 1959; he described 90% satisfactory results but with only short-term follow-up. Hattrup and Johnson[7] popularized the use of the cheilectomy in contemporary practice.

Surgical Technique

This surgical technique was originally published by Mann and colleagues in 1979.[9] A well-illustrated version was published more recently in 2004.[10] The only modification in 25 years was the recommendation to obtain at least 70° of dorsiflexion intraoperatively (rather than 45°). A dorsal longitudinal incision is centered over the MTP joint and is deepened through the capsule on the medial aspect of the extensor hallucis longus tendon. The capsule is preserved for later repair. Hypertrophic synovial tissue and loose bodies are removed from the joint, and the percentage of viable cartilage remaining on the metatarsal head is estimated. The proximal phalanx is plantar flexed, exposing the metatarsal head. An osteotome is used to remove the dorsal, medial, and lateral osteophytes along with the dorsal 25% to 33% of the metatarsal head (**Fig. 3**). This resection is begun just dorsal to the edge of the remaining viable metatarsal head articular cartilage; in cases of more severe arthritis, a more extensive metatarsal head resection is performed. Resection of more than 40% of the head is discouraged because of the risk of dorsal subluxation. If less than 50% of the articular surface is viable, cheilectomy is contraindicated and joint ablative procedures should

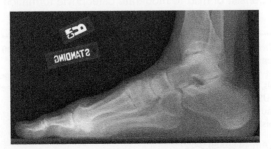

Fig. 1. Lateral weight-bearing radiograph demonstrates hallux rigidus with a large dorsal exostosis of the first metatarsal.

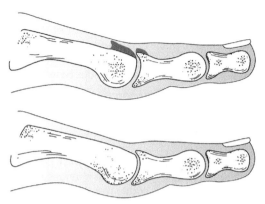

Fig. 2. Diagrammatic representation of a cheilectomy.

be considered, such as arthrodesis. At least 70° of dorsiflexion should be achieved intraoperatively. The osteophytes are then removed from the dorsal aspect of the base of the proximal phalanx. Bone wax may be applied to the cut surface of the metatarsal head. The capsule is repaired beneath the extensor hallucis longus tendon and the skin is closed. Early postoperative range of motion is encouraged to retain the intraoperative gain in motion.

Long-term follow-up data were published in 1979 by Mann and colleagues.[9] They reported a series of 20 patients who underwent cheilectomy for hallux rigidus with a mean follow-up of 67.6 months. Only 3 patients complained of minimal

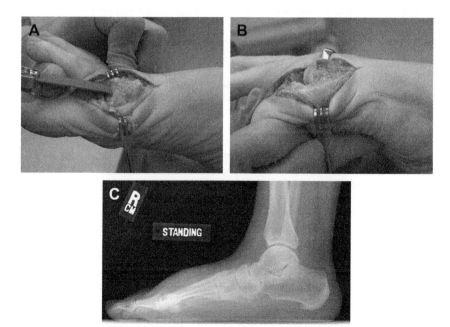

Fig. 3. Cheilectomy. (*A*) First metatarsal dorsal exostosis. (*B*) After resection of the exostosis and the dorsal metatarsal head. (*C*) Postoperative lateral radiograph demonstrates the bony resection.

postoperative discomfort. They ensured at least 45° of dorsiflexion intraoperatively after resection. Postoperatively, patients averaged 30° of dorsiflexion. Preoperative range of motion was not reported. Mann and Clanton[11] reported a series of 28 patients treated with isolated cheilectomy over a 6-year period. Average follow-up was 56 months, with only 3 patients being lost to follow-up. Ninety percent of the patients had less than 30° of dorsiflexion preoperatively, 90% experienced complete pain relief or had minimal residual discomfort, and 74% of patients experienced improvement in their postoperative range of motion, with 68% possessing more than 30° of dorsiflexion. Gould[12] reported a case series of 12 patients treated by cheilectomy who had an average postoperative dorsiflexion of 32°. He stated that all patients were satisfied, although he described the intraoperative findings as "thick pearly, white and adequate cartilage," likely reflecting the relatively low-grade changes in this population.

The previous studies have shown favorable results but did not stratify the patients based on the severity of their arthritis. Several authors have shown less satisfying outcomes with advanced disease states.[7,13] Hattrup and Johnson[7] reviewed 58 cheilectomies in 53 patients with an average follow-up of 37.7 months. Fifty-three percent of the procedures were considered satisfactory, 19% were satisfactory with reservations, and 27.6% were considered unsatisfactory. When the results were correlated with the radiographic appearance of the joint, they found 15% unsatisfactory outcomes with grade I disease, 31.8% with grade II, and 37.5% with grade III. The authors concluded that cheilectomy is a reasonable option for grade I disease but reserved arthrodesis for grades II and III.

Easley and colleagues[13] described a dorsal cheilectomy through a medial approach. They reviewed their series of 52 patients (68 feet) with a minimum 3-year follow-up (mean 63 months). They reported a 90% satisfaction rate. American Orthopaedic Foot and Ankle Society hallux rating scores improved from a preoperative average of 45 points to 85 points at follow-up. Average dorsiflexion improved from 19° to 39°. Eighty-two percent of the feet were grade I or II at the time of operation, and none progressed to failure or required a subsequent procedure by the last follow-up. Of the 18% that were grade III, 8 ft (67%) had continued symptoms, primarily with pain at the midrange of motion, and 3 ft (25%) required arthrodesis.

Other authors have found good results regardless of the radiographic appearance of the joint. Feltham and colleagues[14] reported on a series of 67 patients who underwent cheilectomy, 57 of whom were available for follow-up at a mean of 65 months. The radiographic severity of disease was not used to determine recommendation for surgery; however, "unrelenting, severe, continuous intra-articular pain, including pain at rest, before activity, or at night" was considered an exclusion criterion. An overall satisfaction rate of 78% was found, with 91% satisfaction rate in patients over age 60. This rate included four patients who required salvage with an arthrodesis (three with grade II changes and one with grade III). They also reported that patients who had preoperative symptoms for longer than 72 months had a higher American Orthopaedic Foot and Ankle Society score postoperatively, suggesting that early surgical intervention does not provide better results.

Mulier and colleagues[15] reviewed 20 high-level athletes with a mean age of 30.9 years who underwent 22 cheilectomies with a mean follow-up of 5 years. They reported 95% good or excellent results with an increase in dorsiflexion from 27° preoperatively to 40° postoperatively. Although several authors cited the fact that 7 of the athletes returned to sports at a lower level, this statistic is somewhat misleading, because only 2 patients cited pain in the hallux as the cause for the diminished level of activity. Lau and Daniels[16] retrospectively reviewed a series of 30 patients treated for grade II or III hallux rigidus with a mean 2-year follow-up. Nineteen patients (24 feet) underwent cheilectomy, and 11 patients (11 feet) underwent interpositional arthroplasty. Eighty-three percent of grade II patients were treated with cheilectomy, whereas 91% of grade III patients were treated with arthroplasty. The surgical procedure for cheilectomy was modified slightly to include a closing wedge Moberg osteotomy of the proximal phalanx if dorsiflexion more than 60° could not be obtained intraoperatively. The cheilectomy group had a higher mean American Orthopaedic Foot and Ankle Society score and a satisfaction rate of 88%.

The largest series of cheilectomies to date was published by Coughlin and Shurnas[17] in 2003. They reported on 110 patients treated surgically for hallux rigidus, 80 of whom (93 feet) underwent cheilectomy with a mean duration of follow-up of 9.6 years. Ninety-two percent of the cheilectomies were considered successful, with a mean improvement in dorsiflexion from 14.5° to 38.4°. Nine patients had midrange intra-articular pain preoperatively but underwent cheilectomy at their request. At final follow-up, five of the patients proceeded to arthrodesis, and the remaining four had either fair or poor subjective outcomes.

Multiple studies have shown excellent clinical and subjective outcomes in mild to moderate cases of hallux rigidus with more than 90% satisfaction rates. Care must be taken to identify patients whose complaints are localized to the dorsal exostosis and have minimal or no pain through the midrange of motion. Many authors reported worse outcomes in this patient population, who are more appropriately treated with various joint-destructive techniques. In a series of 80 patients, the most common complication was a superficial wound infection rate of 6% without any incidence of deep infections, neuritis, hypertrophic scar, or tenodesis of the extensor hallucis longus.[17]

PROXIMAL PHALANGEAL OSTEOTOMY

During ambulation, the essential motion of the hallux during toeoff is dorsiflexion. Hallux rigidus is characterized by a painful limited range of motion of the hallux, with the primary deficiency of dorsiflexion, with some preservation of plantarflexion. Use of osteotomy of the phalanx to place the toe into a more "extended" position resets the arc of motion of the joint to better accommodate the need for dorsiflexion. Bonney and Macnab[5] first described a "greenstick extension osteotomy of the proximal phalanx" in adolescents to place the typically preserved plantarflexion range of motion into a more functional arc (**Fig. 4**). Kessel and Bonney[18] were the first to report a series of patients undergoing this procedure. Ten procedures in nine adolescents

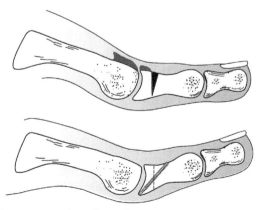

Fig. 4. Diagrammatic representation of a Moberg proximal phalanx osteotomy.

were performed with a mean follow-up of 28 months. Mean dorsiflexion improved from 5° to 44°. All but one patient had relief of pain, and functional activity was restored. They also performed the procedure on a 46-year-old milkman who returned to full-time work at 10 weeks postoperatively, which suggested that the procedure also may be useful in adult patients with established hallux rigidus. Moberg[19] expanded on this theory and published a small series on adults treated with a proximal phalanx extension osteotomy. He performed the operation on eight patients and stated that the results were satisfactory with short-term follow-up. He noted that this report was not a recommendation but rather "a stimulus for further testing."

Surgical Technique

A dorsal approach is often used for this procedure. The incision extends from the inter-phalangeal joint to 1 cm proximal to the first MTP joint. The dorsal periosteum is elevated sharply from the proximal phalanx. Preoperatively, the size of the dorsal wedge is calculated to allow 30° of dorsiflexion of the hallux in relation to the meta-tarsal shaft (15° compared with the plantar surface of the foot). Care must be taken to remove the wedge distal to the epiphysis in adolescent patients. If wire or suture is used to secure the osteotomy, drill holes can be placed before removing the wedge of bone. The plantar cortex remains intact and acts as a hinge for the osteotomy. Kirschner wires or a staple may alternatively be used for fixation (**Fig. 5**). When combined with a cheilectomy, it is imperative to use stable fixation for the osteotomy, because early aggressive range of motion is important in the postoperative period to obtain good results with a cheilectomy.

The first long-term follow-up data were published by Citron and Neil[20] in 1987. They reported on eight patients (10 feet) who underwent dorsal wedge osteotomy of the proximal phalanx with a minimum follow-up of 10 years (mean 22 years). They reported complete pain relief in all patients postoperatively; however, only five joints remained painless at the final follow-up. Only one patient necessitated arthrodesis by the final follow-up. The authors noted progression of arthritis in 90% of the patients at the last follow-up but noted that it "did not correspond with the clinical findings, and most patients remained asymptomatic." Southgate and Urry[21] presented a compar-ison of proximal phalanx dorsal wedge osteotomy to arthrodesis with a mean follow-up of 12 years. Ten osteotomies and 20 arthrodeses were reviewed. No statis-tical comparisons were made, but the authors found similar success in terms of pain relief. The osteotomy group had more complications, more callosities, and greater alterations in foot pressures.

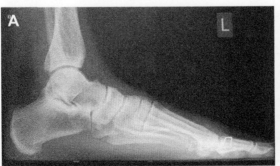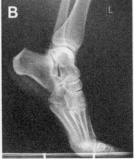

Fig. 5. Moberg proximal phalanx osteotomy. (*A*) Postoperative lateral radiograph. (*B*) Note the significant dorsiflexion achieved at the MTP joint.

Several authors have reported on the use of a dorsal wedge osteotomy in conjunction with a cheilectomy. Blyth and colleagues[22] reviewed a series of 18 patients with a mean follow-up of 4 years. They reported 78% good or excellent results with only one failure that proceeded to arthrodesis. Thomas and Smith[23] published a review of 17 patients (24 feet) with grade I or II disease who underwent a combined procedure. Mean follow-up was 5.2 years. Ninety-six percent of the patients reported that they would undergo the procedure again, with 58% reporting no pain and 42% complaining of mild pain only. Surprisingly, the average increase in dorsiflexion was only 7°. The authors felt that the vast improvement in satisfaction with the combined procedure, compared with cheilectomy alone (96% versus 73% in their series), was not caused by an increase in motion but rather that the dorsal aspect of the joint was decompressed by tilting the proximal phalanx articular surface away from the diseased portion of the metatarsal head. Complications are rare, with two series reporting no adverse outcomes and a single series reporting one nonunion and malunion in ten patients.[19–21]

Osteotomy of the proximal phalanx is rarely indicated as an isolated intervention for hallux rigidus. Evidence demonstrating the efficacy of the Moberg osteotomy in conjunction with a cheilectomy is limited by small patient numbers with limited follow-up. Further studies comparing cheilectomy with and without a Moberg osteotomy are required to delineate the role and use of this osteotomy.

DISTAL METATARSAL OSTEOTOMY

Proponents of metatarsal osteotomies claim that they provide relief from hallux rigidus by either correcting a structural problem with the first ray (excessive length or metatarsus primus elevatus) or by reorienting the proximal portion of the first MTP joint to provide a more functional range of motion. Coughlin and Shurnas[17] demonstrated in a series of 120 patients with hallux rigidus that 94% of the study population had a normal amount of metatarus elevatus. Numerous joint-sparing osteotomies have been described, with differing designs, techniques, and results.

Watermann[24] described a dorsal closing wedge trapezoidal osteotomy of the distal metaphysis of the first metatarsal in 1927. The goal is to orient intact articular cartilage on the plantar surface of the metatarsal head into a more functional position (**Fig. 6**). The dorsal exostosis of the metatarsal head is removed as part of the osteotomy, which in effect produces a cheilectomy. This approach complicates interpreting the

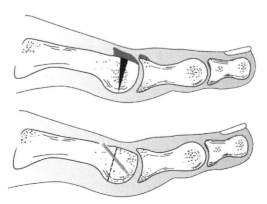

Fig. 6. Diagrammatic representation of a Modified Watermann metatarsal osteotomy.

results, because it is impossible to determine what improvement results from reorientation of the joint surface alone. Cavolo and colleagues[25] reported on two cases treated with this technique. The first patient obtained an increase of 20° to 30° of dorsiflexion and was satisfied. The other patient subjectively had a good outcome, but no objective data were presented to substantiate this claim. The second patient also underwent bilateral proximal metatarsal plantarflexion osteotomies to correct metatarsus primus elevatus, which further confounded the clinical results. Unfortunately, no controlled studies—or even large case series—exist in the literature to adequately validate this technique.

Youngswick[26] described a modification to the Austin (chevron-type) distal osteotomy used for hallux valgus (**Fig. 7**). Treating metatarsus primus elevatus as the root cause of hallux rigidus, his aim was to plantarflex the first metatarsal head to restore more normal joint mechanics. In this modification, after the V-shaped osteotomy is performed, a second osteotomy is made parallel to the dorsal limb, which allows the metatarsal head to translate plantarward, decompressing the joint and eliminating any dorsal impingement. Complications can include fracture, delayed union, and excessive metatarsal shortening. Ten procedures were performed over a 2-year period, but no outcome data were reported. Oloff and Jhala-Patel[27] performed a retrospective analysis of the Youngswick osteotomy when used for late-stage hallux rigidus. Twenty-three patients (28 feet) were selected from a 10-year period based on the severity of their disease and the ability to return for re-evaluation. The mean duration of follow-up was 5.7 years. No objective measures were used in their analysis. Eighty-five percent of patients reported that they were pleased with their outcome, with 75% of those patients reporting more than 90% improvement in their symptoms.

Ronconi and colleagues[28] reviewed a series of patients who underwent a distal oblique osteotomy of the first metatarsal, which shortens the first ray and translates the metatarsal head plantarward (**Fig. 8**). Thirty procedures were performed on 26 patients with a mean follow-up of 21 months. Dorsiflexion improved from 22° to 45°, and 84% of patients reported good or excellent results. The authors noted an increase in the number of patients with pain and excessive pressure under the lesser metatarsal heads and a mean decrease in forefoot supination, both likely because of iatrogenic shortening of the first ray. Gonzalez and colleagues[29] used a similar type of osteotomy to provide plantarflexion of the first metatarsal head. They described a series of 22 patients (25 feet) with a mean follow-up of 12 months. They reported 96% excellent subjective outcomes, with the other patient reporting a good outcome. Mean

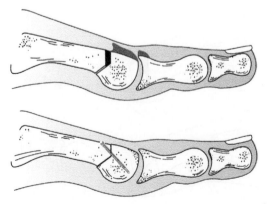

Fig. 7. Diagrammatic representation of a Youngswick chevron metatarsal osteotomy.

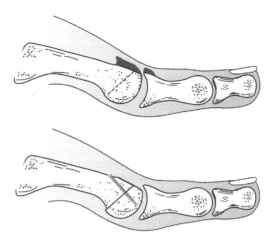

Fig. 8. Diagrammatic representation of a proximal plantar displacement metatarsal osteotomy.

dorsiflexion improved from 18° to 59°. Despite the objective increase in motion, 7 patients (28%) reported a subjective limitation in first MTP joint motion. Two patients complained of sesamoid pain, and no comment was made regarding lesser metatarsalgia. Further follow-up is required to demonstrate if the impressive increase in dorsiflexion is maintained over time.

Derner and colleagues[30] described an alternate plantarflexion-shortening osteotomy of the first metatarsal **(Fig. 9)**. It involves a complete osteotomy perpendicular to the metatarsal shaft and a second parallel, incomplete osteotomy of the distal fragment to create a plantar shelf. The distal fragment is then translated plantar and proximal before being secured. They performed a retrospective review of 26 patients (33 feet) with a mean follow-up of 34.4 months. They reported 85% very good or excellent results, with a mean increase in total range of motion from 33.5° to 72.1°. Improvement in dorsiflexion alone was not measured. Four patients (15%) reported lesser metatarsalgia, with one requiring a second metatarsal shortening; an additional patient reported sesamoid pain.

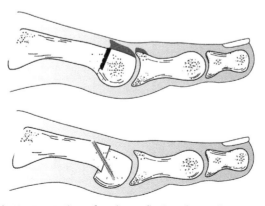

Fig. 9. Diagrammatic representation of a plantarflexion-shortening metatarsal osteotomy.

Roukis and colleagues[31] prospectively evaluated 47 patients (50 feet) who underwent various distal metatarsal decompressive osteotomies with a follow-up of 1 year. Subjectively, 92% of patients stated that they would undergo the procedure again. Postoperative dorsiflexion improved by approximately 6°. Their radiographic interpretation showed significant worsening of the lateral talar-first metatarsal angle, progressive medialization of the second digit, and persistent metatarsus primus elevates, which they felt were secondary to iatrogenic shortening of the first metatarsal with resultant instability of the medial column. This finding was supported clinically by the lack of improvement in two patients with callus under the second metatarsal head and six additional feet that developed new callus.

Kilmartin[32] also performed one of the few prospective, comparative studies in the field by comparing phalangeal osteotomy to distal first metatarsal osteotomy. One hundred eight patients were consecutively enrolled, with the first 49 undergoing phalangeal osteotomy and the remaining 59 undergoing one of three different distal metatarsal osteotomies. Mean follow-up was 29 months for the phalangeal group and 15 months for the metatarsal group. In the phalangeal group, 65% of patients were completely satisfied, 24% were satisfied with reservations, and 11% were dissatisfied. There was no difference in dorsiflexion postoperatively. In the first metatarsal osteotomy group, 54% of patients were completely satisfied, 14% were satisfied with reservations, and 32% were dissatisfied. The mean increase in dorsiflexion was 6°. Eighteen patients (31%) developed transfer metatarsalgia, with six requiring a lesser metatarsal shortening osteotomy. Four patients developed stress fractures of the second metatarsal. The Reverdin-Green osteotomy (**Fig. 10**) was used for this cohort but was abandoned because of the high complication rate. Their conclusion was that neither procedure could be considered definitive for hallux rigidus.

Many of the distal metatarsal osteotomies aim to correct metatarsus primus elevatus and excessively long first metatarsals, resulting in shortening and plantarflexion of the first ray. This result has been shown in many studies to cause significant rates of sesamoiditis, transfer metatarsalgia, and first ray instability. Satisfaction rates are reported as high; however, the high likelihood of complications may lead to diminished returns over time. The proper role for metatarsal osteotomies in the treatment of hallux rigidus remains to be determined.

PROXIMAL METATARSAL OSTEOTOMY

Proximal metatarsal osteotomies also have been described to correct severe cases of metatarsus primus elevatus. As with all angular correction osteotomies, a more

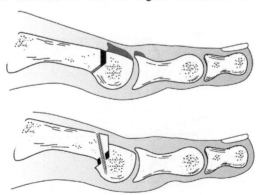

Fig. 10. Diagrammatic representation of a modified Reverdin-Green metatarsal osteotomy.

proximal location provides a more powerful correction. Viegas[33] described a sagittal "Z" osteotomy of the first metatarsal that allows for plantarflexion to correct metatarsus primus elevatus and shortening to correct for a congenitally long first metatarsal (**Fig. 11**). He reported on 11 patients with a mean follow-up of 23 months. All patients had good or excellent outcomes with no pain or restriction in activities. Advantages of this osteotomy include the high cross-sectional area for healing and the ability to use bicortical screw fixation, although the diaphyseal location may result in slower healing rates. Careful review of the surgical technique reveals that before the osteotomy, a full cheilectomy with removal of the dorsal third of the metatarsal head, removal of periarticular osteophytes from the proximal phalanx, mobilization of the soft tissues, and manipulation of the joint is performed. This approach makes it difficult to determine if the favorable outcomes result from the osteotomy or the cheilectomy.

Drago and colleagues[34] described a modified sagittal Logroscino osteotomy that combines the distal closing wedge osteotomy of Watermann with a proximal plantarflexion opening wedge osteotomy (**Fig. 12**). This procedure combines the ability to rotate the distal cartilage into a more functional position with correction of the metatarsus primus elevatus. The authors suggested that it should be used only in younger patients when no evidence of cartilage degeneration is seen. No clinical data were provided to substantiate the "excellent functional and clinical result" they reported.

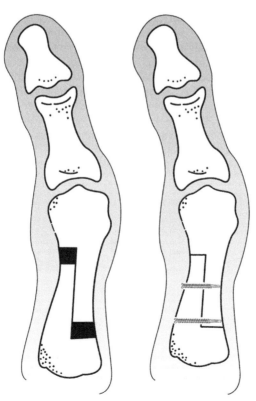

Fig. 11. Diagrammatic representation of a sagittal "Z" metatarsal osteotomy.

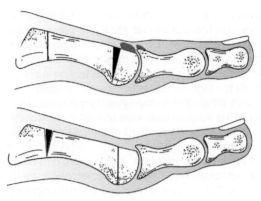

Fig. 12. Diagrammatic representation of a sagittal Logroscino metatarsal osteotomies.

Postoperative hallux MTP motion is also a concern because they stated that this procedure "requires at least six weeks of below-the-knee cast immobilization."

OTHER PROCEDURES

A sagittal plane "V" resection of the first MTP joint, termed the Valenti procedure, has been described in the podiatric literature (**Fig. 13**). Grady and Axe[35] reported on 21 patients, citing improved pain scores and a mean improvement in dorsiflexion of 12°. Saxena[36] was able to achieve superior postoperative motion. He described 11 patients (12 feet) with a mean follow-up of 21 months. Dorsiflexion improved by 27°. Nine patients reported good or excellent results. Kurtz and colleagues[37] provided long-term data on the Valenti procedure. Thirty-three patients (36 feet) were evaluated at a mean of 4.1 years. Thirty-three of the procedures had a good or excellent outcome based on a written survey. Only 8 patients (11 feet) were available for examination. A mean of 45° of dorsiflexion was achieved in that small group. This procedure may be an alternative to resection arthroplasty when the disease process is too advanced for a cheilectomy and the patient is a poor candidate for arthrodesis.

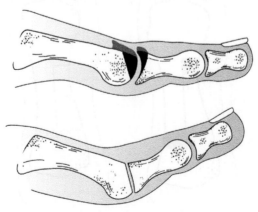

Fig. 13. Diagrammatic representation of a Valenti procedure.

SUMMARY

Cheilectomy remains the gold standard of treatment for mild to moderate hallux rigidus. Long-term follow-up of large groups of patients has demonstrated excellent results. The literature is also replete with metatarsal and phalangeal osteotomies for the correction of proposed underlying causes of hallux rigidus. A cheilectomy to remove the offending dorsal osteophytes is included in most of these procedures, however, which confounds interpretation of the results from these osteotomies. These procedures may confer other benefits; however, they add the risks of nonunion and malunion and may create secondary deformities or instability. These complications must be weighed when considering these procedures. Recent studies also have not demonstrated an association between hallux rigidus and metatarsus elevatus or a long first metatarsal. Further investigation demonstrating a definitive causal relationship is required before endorsing the widespread use of these procedures that purportedly seek to correct those deformities.

REFERENCES

1. Davies-Colley M. Contraction of the metatarsophalangeal joint of the great toe. BMJ 1887;1:728.
2. Cotterill JM. Stiffness of the great toe in adolescents. BMJ 1888;1:158.
3. McMaster MJ. The pathogenesis of hallux rigidus. J Bone Joint Surg Br 1978; 60(1):82–7.
4. Nilsonne H. Hallux rigidus and its treatment. Acta Orthop Scand 1930;1:295–303.
5. Bonney G, Macnab I. Hallux valgus and hallux rigidus: a critical survey of operative results. J Bone Joint Surg Br 1952;34(3):366–85.
6. Lambrinudi C. Metatarsus primus elevatus. Proc R Soc Med 1938;31:1273.
7. Hattrup SJ, Johnson KA. Subjective results of hallux rigidus following treatment with cheilectomy. Clin Orthop Relat Res 1988;226:182–91.
8. DuVries HV. Static deformities. In: DuVries HV, editor. Surgery of the foot. St. Louis (MO): Mosby Year Book; 1959. p. 392–9.
9. Mann RA, Coughlin MJ, DuVries HL, et al. Hallux rigidus: a review of the literature and a method of treatment. Clin Orthop Relat Res 1979;142:57–63.
10. Coughlin MJ, Shurnas PS. Hallux rigidus: surgical techniques (cheilectomy and arthrodesis). J Bone Joint Surg Am 2004;86:119–30.
11. Mann RA, Clanton TO. Hallux rigidus: treatment by cheilectomy. J Bone Joint Surg Am 1988;70(3):400–6.
12. Gould N. Hallux rigidus: cheilectomy or implant? Foot Ankle 1981;1(6):315–20.
13. Easley ME, Davis WH, Anderson RB. Intermediate to long-term follow-up of medial-approach dorsal cheilectomy for hallux rigidus. Foot Ankle Int 1999; 20(3):147–52.
14. Feltham GT, Hanks SE, Marcus RE, et al. Age-based outcomes of cheilectomy for the treatment of hallux rigidus. Foot Ankle Int 2001;22(3):192–7.
15. Mulier T, Steenwerckx A, Thienpont E, et al. Results after cheilectomy in athletes with hallux rigidus. Foot Ankle Int 1999;20(4):232–7.
16. Lau JT, Daniels TR. Outcomes following cheilectomy and interpositional arthroplasty in hallux rigidus. Foot Ankle Int 2001;22(6):462–70.
17. Coughlin MJ, Shurnas PJ. Hallux rigidus: grading and long-term results of operative treatment. J Bone Joint Surg Am 2003;85(11):2072–88.
18. Kessel L, Bonney G. Hallux rigidus in the adolescent. J Bone Joint Surg Br 1958; 40(4):668–73.

19. Moberg E. A simple operation for hallux rigidus. Clin Orthop Relat Res 1979;142: 55–6.
20. Citron N, Neil M. Dorsal wedge osteotomy of the proximal phalanx for hallux rigidus: long-term results. J Bone Joint Surg Br 1987;69(5):835–7.
21. Southgate JJ, Urry SR. Hallux rigidus: the long-term results of dorsal wedge osteotomy and arthrodesis in adults. J Foot Ankle Surg 1997;36(2):136–40.
22. Blyth MJ, Mackay DC, Kinninmonth AW, et al. Dorsal wedge osteotomy in the treatment of hallux rigidus. J Foot Ankle Surg 1998;37(1):8–10.
23. Thomas PJ, Smith RW. Proximal phalanx osteotomy for the surgical treatment of hallux rigidus. Foot Ankle Int 1999;20(1):3–12.
24. Watermann H. Die arthritis deformans des großzehen-grundgelenkes als selbständiges krankheitsbild. Z Orthop Chir 1927;48:346–55.
25. Cavolo DJ, Cavallaro DC, Arrington LE, et al. The Watermann osteotomy for hallux limitus. J Am Podiatry Assoc 1979;69:52–7.
26. Youngswick FD. Modifications of the Austin bunionectomy for treatment of metatarsus primus elevatus associated with hallux limitus. J Foot Surg 1982;21:114–6.
27. Oloff LM, Jhala-Patel G. A retrospective analysis of joint salvage procedures for grades III and IV hallux rigidus. J Foot Ankle Surg 2008;47(3):230–6.
28. Ronconi P, Monachino P, Baleanu PM, et al. Distal oblique osteotomy of the first metatarsal for the correction of hallux limitus and rigidus deformity. J Foot Ankle Surg 2000;39(3):154–60.
29. Gonzalez JV, Garrett PP, Jordan MJ, et al. The modified Hohmann osteotomy: an alternative joint salvage procedure for hallux rigidus. J Foot Ankle Surg 2004; 43(6):380–8.
30. Derner R, Goss K, Postowski HN, et al. A plantarflexory-shortening osteotomy for hallux rigidus: a retrospective analysis. J Foot Ankle Surg 2005;44(5):377–89.
31. Roukis TS, Jacobs PM, Dawson DM, et al. A prospective comparison of clinical, radiographic, and intraoperative features of hallux rigidus: short-term follow-up and analysis. J Foot Ankle Surg 2002;41(3):158–65.
32. Kilmartin TE. Phalangeal osteotomy versus first metatarsal decompression osteotomy for the surgical treatment of hallux rigidus: a prospective study of age-matched and condition-matched patients. J Foot Ankle Surg 2005;44(1):2–12.
33. Viegas GV. Reconstruction of hallux limitus deformity using a first metatarsal sagittal-Z osteotomy. J Foot Ankle Surg 1998;37(3):204–11.
34. Drago JJ, Oloff L, Jacobs AM, et al. A comprehensive review of hallux limitus. J Foot Surg 1984;23(3):213–20.
35. Grady JF, Axe TM. The modified Valenti procedure for the treatment of hallux limitus. J Foot Ankle Surg 1994;33(4):365–7.
36. Saxena A. The Valenti procedure for hallux limitus/rigidus. J Foot Ankle Surg 1995;34(5):485–8.
37. Kurtz DH, Harrill JC, Kaczander BI, et al. The Valenti procedure for hallux limitus: a long-term follow-up and analysis. J Foot Ankle Surg 1999;38(2):123–30.

Hallux Rigidus: Surgical Treatment with the Crescentic Oblique Basilar Resection Arthroplasty (COBRA)

Richard M. Marks, MD, FACS

KEYWORDS

- Hallux rigidus • Hallux valgus
- First metatarsophalangeal arthritis • Resection arthroplasty

Hallux rigidus, defined as painful, restricted, dorsal motion of the hallux, is associated with proliferative osteophytic bone formation on the dorsal aspect of the joint, with resultant loss of dorsiflexion. This condition may simply restrict hallux dorsiflexion because of dorsal bony impingement, or in more severe cases, include global arthritis of the first metatarsophalangeal joint. The etiology of hallux rigidus is multifactorial in origin. An adolescent form of hallux rigidus includes localized changes in the dorsal–central cartilage that represents more of an osteochondral defect picture. The adult type is multifactorial in origin. The etiology of the adult type most commonly is post-traumatic, either following fracture about the joint, or from repetitive trauma to the joint, frequently subacute in nature. Other causes include idiopathic, inflammatory, and structural abnormalities, such as congenital flattening or squaring off of the metatarsal head, which may lead to increased stresses across the dorsal aspect of the joint. Relative dorsiflexion of the first metatarsal relative to the proximal phalanx also may predispose an individual to increased dorsal stresses on the articular cartilage of the first metatarsal head.

The end result of the altered stresses across the joint is osteophyte formation, typically dorsally and laterally. Dorsal impingement results in pain with any activities that require dorsiflexion of the joint, particularly running, squatting, and climbing stairs. In the early stages of hallux rigidus, this is characterized by sharp discomfort with these activities that is relieved with rest. As the hallux rigidus progresses to more advanced, global arthritis of the joint, pain is not relieved with rest or cessation of causative

Department of Orthopedic Surgery, Division of Foot and Ankle Surgery, Medical College of Wisconsin, 9200 West Wisconsin Avenue, Milwaukee, WI 53226, USA
E-mail address: rmarks@mcw.edu

Foot Ankle Clin N Am 14 (2009) 23–32
doi:10.1016/j.fcl.2008.11.005

foot.theclinics.com

activities necessarily. In more severe cases, proliferative osteophyte formation may create difficulty with footwear, and perhaps ulceration.

TREATMENT OPTIONS
Nonoperative

Nonoperative treatment options include the institution of anti-inflammatory agents, and shoe modifications such as a higher toe box, stiffer sole, and the use of an orthotic with Morton's extension, which stiffens the medial column, thus placing less stress across the first metatarsophalangeal joint. In some instances, a steroid injection may provide relief; however, this frequently is temporary.

Operative

Surgical treatment options are based on the specific pathology and degree of disease. Isolated osteochondral injury is treated with debridement and drilling of the defect, and in larger defects, consideration may be given for placement of an osteochondral plug in the defect. Dorsal joint impingement with a relatively well-preserved joint space is treated with a cheilectomy, which resects 20% to 30% of the articular surface of the first metatarsal head. Dorsal osteophyte recurrence is rare, and few cases require eventual fusion of the joint.

Treatment options for more advanced arthritic changes depend on age, comorbidities, and activity level. Described procedures include fusion of the first metatarsophalangeal joint, resection arthroplasty, and joint replacement, either with total joint replacement, hemi-arthroplasty, or silicone implant. Active patients who have good bone stock and the ability to comply with protected weight bearing in the postoperative period are good candidates for fusion of the joint. Joint replacement or hemi-arthroplasty has been described; however, it does not allow for resumption of high-impact activities and is associated with an unacceptable failure and complication rate.[1]

The remaining option, and the focus of this article, is resection arthroplasty. In 1904,[2] Keller described resection of the proximal one third of the proximal phalanx for treating hallux valgus. Many surgeons adopted this procedure as their treatment for hallux valgus. The resultant complications included a recurrence rate of up to 50%, hallux varus, the development of a cock-up deformity because of destabilization of the plantar plate and supporting structures, and transfer metatarsalgia caused by loss of first ray length, as well as the loss of push-off power (**Fig. 1**).[1,3–7] Additionally, stress fracture of the lesser metatarsals caused by loss of first ray length and load sharing has been reported.[8,9] For this reason, many have abandoned this procedure, not without just cause.

Others have attempted to modify Keller's resection arthroplasty, in an attempt to provide a viable treatment alternative for lower-demand individuals who require correction of their hallux rigidus or hallux valgus deformity without the need for a healing of osteotomies or incorporation of internal fixation. Surgical modifications include the creation of an interpositional arthroplasty using the extensor hallucis brevis,[10] volar plate mobilization with medial capsule placation,[11] extensor hallucis brevis (EHB) transfer to the medial sesamoid combined with a molded arthroplasty,[12] a crescentic basilar resection by means of a medial approach,[13] and an oblique dorsal–distal to plantar–proximal resection with interposition of the EHB.[14]

CRESCENTIC OBLIQUE BASILAR RESECTION ARTHROPLASTY

In an attempt to surgically address individuals who have advanced hallux rigidus or hallux valgus but are not candidates for fusion or traditional hallux valgus correction,

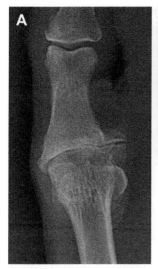
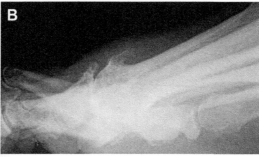

Fig.1. (*A*) Cock-up and varus deformity status post Keller, with (*B*) Radiographic appearance.

a unique approach to correction of these deformities has been developed. Indications for the crescentic oblique basilar resection arthroplasty (COBRA) procedure include:

Advanced hallux rigidus with arthritis in elderly, low-demand population
Advanced hallux valgus in elderly, low-demand population
Advanced hallux rigidus/valgus with poor bone stock
Advanced hallux rigidus with arthritis in patients unwilling to undergo fusion

Recognizing that the drawbacks of the traditional Keller resection arthroplasty and its modifications include shortening of the hallux with risk of metatarsalgia and stress fracture, disruption of the plantar soft tissues with the potential for loss of push-off strength, and development of cock-up deformity, COBRA has been developed. This procedure entails a dorsal incision, with resection of the base of the proximal phalanx using a crescentic saw blade, oriented from a dorsal–distal to plantar–proximal direction, with the saw blade exiting just distal to the base of the proximal phalanx to maintain the plantar plate and maximize hallux length (**Fig. 2**). The crescentic saw blade also creates a congruent surface at the base of the phalanx that matches the first metatarsal head. A transverse resection would result in a concentration of stresses on the central aspect of the first metatarsal head. The dorsal incision also allows for release of the contracted lateral soft tissues in the case of hallux valgus and resection of the medial eminence. In cases of advanced hallux rigidus, a cheilectomy can be performed through the dorsal incision.

SURGICAL TECHNIQUE

The procedure typically is performed under an ankle block with intravenous sedation. The patient is placed supine on the operating table and prepared to midcalf. An Esmarch bandage is used to exsanguinate the foot and ankle, then used as a tourniquet at the supramalleolar level.

A longitudinal incision is performed just medial to the extensor hallucis longus (EHL) tendon, and carried down to the level of the capsule, which is entered sharply (**Fig. 3**A). Dorsal and lateral osteophytes are removed with a rongeur. The base of the proximal

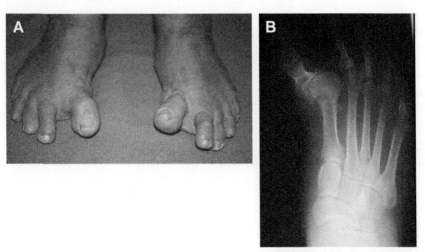

Fig. 2. (*A*) Loss of joint space, sclerosis, and medial and lateral ostophytes associated with advanced hallux rigidus. (*B*) Lateral radiograph showing lipping dorsal osteophyte and loss of joint space.

phalanx is mobilized sufficiently to allow Homann retractors to be placed at the base of the phalanx for the resection arthroplasty. Care must be taken to avoid destabilization of the plantar soft tissues.

In cases with concomitant hallux valgus, the medial eminence is resected with a chisel and mallet, and a laminar spreader placed in the first dorsal web space to allow for release of the adductor hallucis, intermetatarsal ligament, and lateral capsule. If there is associated EHL tendon contracture that tethers the hallux laterally, it is lengthened in a Z-fashion. In some cases, the surgeon can wait until the oblique resection arthroplasty is performed and the esmarch is released to reassess the lateral soft tissue contracture. In cases of isolated hallux rigidus, a formal cheilectomy is performed, resecting the dorsal 15% to 20% of the articular surface (**Fig. 3**B). Because of the oblique basilar resection arthroplasty, less bone needs to be resected compared with a standard cheilectomy. The joint then is checked for any residual impingement.

The basilar resection arthroplasty now is performed with a crescentic saw blade (Stryker, Memphis, Tennessee). The saw blade is oriented from a distal dorsal to plantar–proximal direction (**Fig. 3**C). The proximal 20% of the base of the phalanx is resected, with the saw exiting just dorsal to the plantar base of the phalanx, thereby

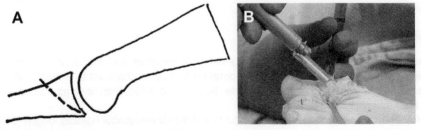

Fig. 3. (*A*) Graphic representation and (*B*) Intra-operative view of dorsal-distal to plantar-proximal crescentic sawblade orientation.

maintaining a small shelf of bone (**Fig. 3**D), which avoids destabilizing the plantar plate. In some large individuals, the radius of curvature of the blade may not match the bony architecture, and a rongeur will need to be used to trim the medial and lateral base of the proximal phalanx. Once completed, the oblique basilar resection should have created a congruent resection surface with the first metatarsal head, and adequately decompressed the joint (**Fig. 3**E,F). The sesamoid complex is not mobilized with this procedure.

The joint is irrigated, and fixation of the COBRA is performed with two 0.062 K-wires placed antegrade out the distal phalanx, then brought proximally across the metatarsophalangeal joint. The hallux is positioned in a corrected position for cases of concomitant hallux valgus, and if there is concern about the possible need for an EHL lengthening, the esmarch is released before this step. An important point is to ensure that the joint is distracted when the K-wires are placed retrograde across the joint (**Fig. 3**G). This distraction ensures proper length restoration after the procedure, and avoids the need for soft tissue interposition.

Closure is performed in three layers, using 2.0 absorbable sutures for the capsule, 3.0 absorbable sutures for the subcutaneous tissues, and 4.0 nylon for skin. The EHL tendon is repaired as indicated. A forefoot dressing is applied in the operating suite.

Postoperative Treatment

Postoperatively, patients are instructed to elevate their foot for the first 10 days; heel weight bearing in a postoperative shoe is allowed. At 10 days, the sutures are removed, and if the soft tissues allow, no further dressing is necessary, given the stability afforded by the K-wires. If the patient is treated primarily for hallux rigidus, the K-wires are removed at 4 weeks, and range-of-motion exercises are instituted with physical therapy. In cases with concomitant hallux valgus, the K-wires remain in for 6 weeks to allow the soft tissue release to scar in and repair. Unlike the younger, more active population that requires maximal restoration of motion, this procedure is performed to achieve angular correction and resolution of arthritic symptoms, with less regard for motion, as all of these joints are quite stiff preoperatively.

I prefer a formal physical therapy program to maximize the use of modalities, and to monitor patient symptoms. Patients also receive a silastic gel strip that is applied daily to minimize scarring of the incision. Vitamin E oil or similar scar emollient also is used. In patients who have preoperative lesser metatarsalgia, an accommodative orthotic with Morton's extension and protection of the lesser metatarsal heads frequently is prescribed.

SURGICAL RESULTS

The COBRA procedure initially was performed in May of 2000. Since then, 52 procedures have been performed in 50 patients. The author previously reported results of our initial 28 procedures, 16 with a minimum of 6 months follow-up.[15] Fifteen women and one man, with a mean age of 73.2 years (range, 59 to 81 years) underwent the COBRA procedure. The diagnosis was hallux rigidus in seven patients, hallux valgus with hallux rigidus in seven, and silastic implant failure in two. Additional procedures performed include hammertoe correction (10), shortening metatarsal osteotomy (3), and metatarsal head resection (8) procedures.

Radiographic evaluation was performed preoperatively and at 6 months follow-up. Radiographs were evaluated for hallux valgus angle (HVA), intermetatarsal angle (IMA), the development of stress reaction or fracture of the lesser metatarsals, and development of hallux varus or cock-up deformity.

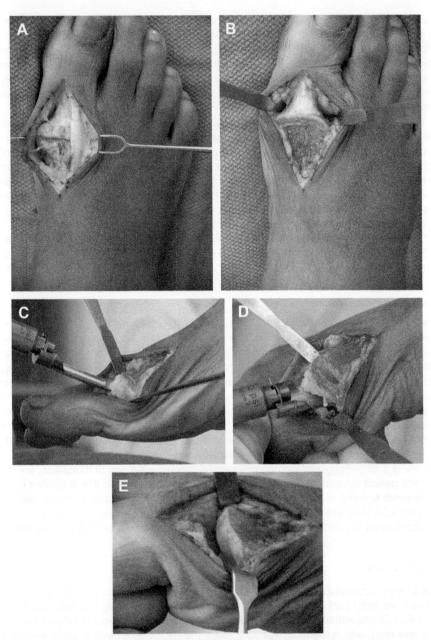

Fig. 4. (*A*) A dorsal incision is made, and the EHL tendon reflected laterally. (*B*) Dorsal chei-lectomy completed. (*C*) The crescentic sawblade is oriented dorsal-distal to plantar-proximal, and (*D*) exits just dorsal to the plantar base and plantar plate. (*E*) Lateral and (*F*) Anteropos-terior (AP) appearance after resection. Note the congruent resection surfaces. (*G*) Kirschner wire (K-wire) fixation with distraction of the joint.

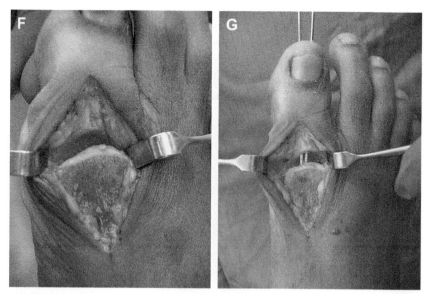

Fig. 4. (*continued*).

Clinical evaluation was performed postoperatively to evaluate for transfer metatarsalgia, plantarflexion strength, and cock-up deformity. Patients also were asked to fill out a satisfaction questionnaire. Specific questions included rating of pain (none, mild, moderate, severe), activity limitations (none, minimal, moderate, severe), footwear

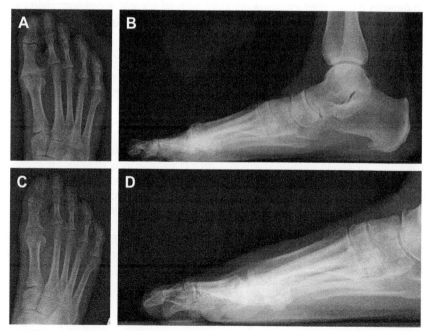

Fig. 5. (*A*) Anteroposterior (AP) and (*B*) lateral pre-operative radiographs. (*C*) AP and (*D*) lateral post-operative radiographs. Note the oblique slope of the resection on the lateral.

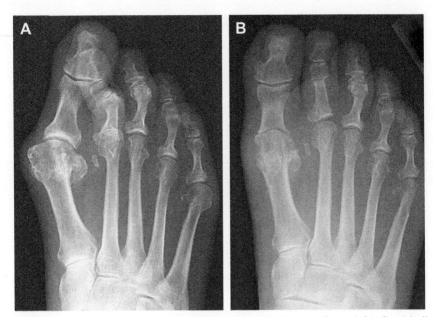

Fig. 6. (*A*) Pre- and (*B*) post-operative radiographs of COBRA performed for fixed hallux valgus deformity.

restrictions, patient satisfaction (completely satisfied, satisfied with minor reservations, satisfied with major reservations, unsatisfied), and if they were willing to undergo the procedure again.

All patients healed their incisions primarily, with no complications associated with the K-wire fixation. The preoperative HVA averaged 33.8°, (range, 19° to 53°). Postoperatively, the HVA averaged 16.4°, (range, 2° to 28°), with an average correction of 17.4°. The preoperative IMA averaged 15.9° (range, 5° to 30°). Postoperatively, the IMA improved to 10.7° (range, 6° to 17°), with an average correction of 5.2° (**Figs. 4–6**).

Postoperatively, patients reported no activity limitations in 75% of cases, and only mild limitations in the other 25%. Pain relief was achieved in 94% of patients, and only one (6.2%) postoperative complication was reported, in an inflammatory arthritis patient who had wound dehiscence that responded to wound care and wound vacuum application with no further sequelae.

There was no case of postoperative transfer metatarsalgia, cock-up deformity, hallux varus, or stress fracture/reaction, with full maintenance of push-off strength. All patients were pleased with their postoperative appearance, and all patients were able to wear normal shoes. Eight patients (50%) wore accommodative orthotics; however, all of these patients required orthotics preoperatively.

Clinical satisfaction rating of the procedure revealed 87.5% (14 of 16 patients) were completely satisfied with the outcome, with two patients (12.5%) satisfied with mild reservations; both of these patients had failed silastic implants. All patients reported that they would undergo the procedure again.

SUMMARY

The treatment of advanced hallux rigidus in an older, more sedentary population with poor bone stock or comorbidities that may make corrective osteotomy, fusion, and implant fixation more problematic has frequently been an issue for orthopedic surgeons. The traditional Keller resection arthroplasty has not fared well because of problems with recurrence, hallux varus, cock-up deformity, and loss of push-off strength. Additionally, the subsequent loss of hallux length has led to transfer metatarsalgia and lesser metatarsal stress fracture, while being cosmetically unsatisfactory.

Although attempts have been made to modify Keller's procedure, none have addressed preservation of the plantar plate, maintenance of hallux length, and the creation of a congruent joint surface at the base of the proximal phalanx. The COBRA procedure, by virtue of the oblique crescentic bone resection, preserves the plantar plate, maintains hallux length, and creates a congruent resection surface for the metatarsal head, thereby avoiding concentration of stresses on the central aspect of the first metatarsal head. Initial results with this procedure have shown an improvement of the HVA by 17.4°, and an improvement of the IMA by 5.2°. No cases of hallux varus, cock-up, transfer metatarsalgia, or stress fracture/reaction have been reported. All patients were satisfied with the procedure and willing to undergo the surgery again. All were able to wear normal shoes after the procedure.

The COBRA is a viable surgical treatment alternative for older, more sedentary patients with advanced hallux rigidus with or without hallux valgus. This may also be a good alternative procedure in a more active patient who wishes to avoid fusion of the joint while maintaining some first metatarsophalangeal joint (MTP) motion. The procedure also avoids the need for harvesting tendon for interpositional arthroplasty or performing a tendon transfer.

REFERENCES

1. Johnson KA, Saltzman CL. Complications of resection arthroplasty (Keller) and replacement arthroplasty (silicone) procedures. Contemp Orthop 1991;23(2): 139–47.
2. Keller WL. The surgical treatment of bunions and hallux valgus. NY Med J 1904; 80:741–2.
3. Belt EA, Kaarela K, Kauppi MJ, et al. Outcome of Keller resection arthroplasty in the rheumatoid foot. A radiographic follow-up study of 4 to 11 years. Clin Exp Rheumatol 1999;17(3):387.
4. Flamme CH, Wulker N, Kuckerts K, et al. Follow-up results 17 years after resection arthroplasty of the great toe. Arch Orthop Trauma Surg 1998;117(8):457–60, Erratum in: Arch Ortho Trauma Surg 1999;119(3–4):243.
5. Fuhrmann RA, Anders JO. The long-term results of resection arthroplasties of the first metatarsophalangeal joint in rheumatoid arthritis. Int Orthop 2001;25(5): 312–6.
6. McGarvey SR, Johnson KA. Keller arthroplasty in combination with resection arthroplasty of the lesser metatarsophalangeal joints in rheumatoid arthritis. Foot Ankle 1988;9(2):75–80.
7. Stewart J, Reed JF 3rd. An audit of Keller arthroplasty and metatarsophalangeal joint arthrodesis from national data. Int J Low Extrem Wounds 2003;2(2):69–73.
8. Danon G, Pokrassa M. An unusual complication of the Keller bunionectomy: spontaneous stress fractures of all lesser metatarsals. J Foot Surg 1989;28(4): 335–9.
9. Ford LT, Gilula LA. Stress fractures of the middle metatarsals following the Keller operation. J Bone Joint Surg Am 1977;59(1):117–8.
10. Hamilton WG, Hubbard CE. Hallux rigidus. Excisional arthroplasty. Foot Ankle Clin 2000;5(3):663–71.
11. Lelievre J. Pathologic du pied. Paris: Masson; 1970. p. 222–6.

12. Capasso G, Testa V, Maffulli N, et al. Molded arthroplasty and transfer of extensor hallucis brevis tendon. A modification of the Keller-Lelievre operation. Clin Orthop Relat Res 1994;(308):43–9.
13. Harper MC. A modified Keller resection arthroplasty. Foot Ankle Int 1995;16(4): 236–7.
14. Mroczek KJ, Miller SD. The modified oblique Keller procedure: a technique for dorsal approach interposition arthroplasty sparing the flexor tendons. Foot Ankle Int 2003;24(7):521–2.
15. Marks RM, Cush G. Treatment of advanced hallux valgus & hallux rigidus with a crescentic oblique basilar resection arthroplasty. Presented at the International Federation of Foot & Ankle Societies, 2nd Joint Meeting of Asian, European, North American, South American Federations. Naples, Italy, September 15–18, 2005.

Hallux Rigidus: MTP Implant Arthroplasty

Martin R. Sullivan, MBBS (Hon), FRACS, FAOrthA

KEYWORDS

- Hallux rigidus • Arthroplasty • Great toe • Joint replacement
- Cheilectomy • Townley hemiarthroplasty

Hallux rigidus or osteoarthritis of the first metatarsophalangeal (MTP) joint is characterized by pain, stiffness of the joint, and alterations of gait. Pain and altered joint mechanics can lead to weight being transferred to the outer border of the foot during gait[1–4] or they can cause one to rotate the hip externally during the swing phase of gait to allow for the toe to clear.[3] Daily activities, such as stair climbing, squatting, walking, and kneeling, can be impaired.[5] For an implant to be effective it should restore joint kinematics, be long lasting, and not be difficult to revise if it fails.

Hallux rigidus involves the loss of articular cartilage and in the severe stages can also involve bone stock loss. This can lead to shortening of the first metatarsal, which has implications in the assessment and surgical treatment of grade 4 hallux rigidus **(Fig. 1)**.[6] The need for a properly constructed, prospective study to develop a suitable classification system for hallux rigidus has been recently highlighted by Beeson and colleagues.[7]

Weight-bearing radiographs should be taken and the relative length of the first metatarsal assessed because further shortening of the first metatarsal either with an arthrodesis or arthroplasty can alter the mechanics leading to pathologic overload of the second metatarsal, relative lengthening of the second metatarsal, and tearing of the plantar plate of the second metatarsal resulting in pain. Transfer metatarsalgia has been described following surgery for hallux rigidus either with an arthrodesis or arthroplasty.

INDICATIONS AND CONTRAINDICATIONS

Coughlin and Shumas[8] in a long-term study over 19 years of patients with hallux rigidus indicated the average age at onset of symptoms was 43 years and the average age at surgery was 50 years. Hallux rigidus involves a younger, active group seeking alternatives to arthrodesis. Early stage hallux rigidus is typically approached by joint debridement and cheilectomy. Metatarsal and phalangeal osteotomies have also been described.[9]

St. Vincent's Clinic, Suite 901E, 438 Victoria Street, Sydney, Australia 2010
E-mail address: drmsullivan@hotmail.com

Foot Ankle Clin N Am 14 (2009) 33–42
doi:10.1016/j.fcl.2008.11.009
1083-7515/08/$ – see front matter © 2009 Elsevier Inc. All rights reserved.

foot.theclinics.com

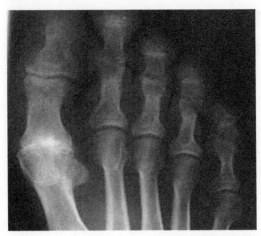

Fig.1. Grade 4 hallux rigidus with bone stock loss predominantly laterally and relative shortening of the first metatarsal.

Arthrodesis of the first MTP joint eliminates painful motion of the whole joint including the sesamoid-metatarsal articulation and is associated with a predictable outcome in terms of pain relief. It can lead, however, to progressive arthritis of the interphalangeal joint[10–15] and nonunion rates of up to 10% have been reported.[16,17] Arthrodesis produces stiffness of the toe and has impact on gait.

Arthrodesis of the first MTP joint was assessed by Defrino and colleagues[1] using dynamic pedobarography. Their results demonstrated restoration of weight-bearing on the first ray with greater force carried by the great toe at toe-off. For patients with a relatively short first metatarsal there is a risk of load transfer to the lesser metatarsal heads after arthrodesis. There is also a reduction in ankle plantar flexion at toe-off on the arthrodesed side. The loss of dorsiflexion maybe an issue for certain occupations that require kneeling or squatting, in runners, and in women who feel the need to wear high heels.

Such concerns have heightened interest in hallux MTP joint replacement. The appeal of joint arthroplasty for hallux rigidus is similar to its benefits in other joints in the body. The ideal implant should relieve pain, restore motion, improve function, and maintain joint stability. It should be salvageable if it fails.[18] Implant arthroplasty should improve the altered kinematics of the first MTP joint and restore weight bearing of the hallux. Implant durability is also a desirable feature.

Numerous implants have been described for the hallux MTP joint. This article discusses various implant options along with clinical outcomes and complications.

SILASTIC IMPLANTS

The results of Silastic implants used in the great toe were first published 30 years ago.[19] The Silastic implants are designed to maintain length of the toe and act as a dynamic spacer, which allows the joint to move. Cracchiolo and coworkers[20] published in 1992, with average 6-year follow-up, the outcome showing there was an average range of motion of 42 degrees in the first MTP joint; however, the implant fractured in 10% of cases and cystic formation was noted on the radiographs of one third of the patients. This suggested that the implants may not be durable and that the incidence of patients requiring revision surgery was likely to increase. Later, the design of the implant was altered and titanium grommets were inserted to aid the survival of the implant.[21,22] Unfortunately, reports followed by Granberry and coworkers[23] indicating fracture of the implant was related to the duration of implantation particularly after 4 years. The incidence of osteolysis and possible pathologic fracture increases with time. Along with this implant failure, bone stock loss can lead to significant shortening of the first ray causing a cock-up deformity of the great toe and transfer metatarsalgia with eventual dislocation of the second MTP joint (**Figs. 2** and **3**).

It is possible to salvage patients who have had failed Silastic implants inserted. It is well recognized[24] that patients can have implant fracture and severe osteolysis with a lack of symptoms. It is possible for patients with long-standing implants to present with sudden onset of pain caused by pathologic fracture of the osteolytic bone. Previously, to salvage this involved a large bone graft and formal arthrodesis.[24] Kitaoka and coworkers,[25] however, reported good to excellent results by removing the implant and performing a thorough synovectomy and debridement of the bone.

The use of Silastic implants is, however, associated with many reported complications.[26–33] Failure of the implant because of wear, early fracture of the implant, dislodgement of the implant, Silastic synovitis and osteolysis, and silicone debris causing foreign body reactions have been reported. The possibility of systemic invasion of the lymphatic system with silicone microparticles is also a major concern,[34–36] and the presence of inguinal lymph node foreign body granulomas after a silicone implant was implanted in the great toe has been described in 1996.

HEMIARTHROPLASTY: PHALANGEAL, METATARSAL

The use of metal as a surface replacement was described by Townley and Taranow[37] in 1994 and was first used in the 1950s. The Biopro (Biopro, Port Huron, Michigan) hemiarthroplasty is a cobalt-chrome alloy resurfacing prosthesis for the proximal phalanx of the great toe. It allows for minimal bone resection (2 mm), which can

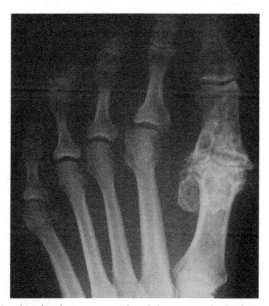

Fig. 2. The Silastic implant has been removed and there is marked relative shortening of the first metatarsal.

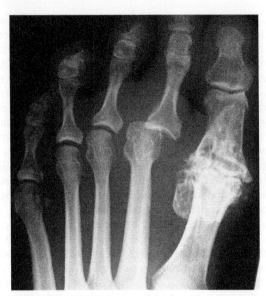

Fig. 3. The second metatarsophalangeal joint is now dislocated causing transfer metatarsalgia.

maintain length of the great toe and does not interfere with the muscle attachments to the proximal phalanx.[38] Townley implanted 312 prostheses over a span of 40 years. He reported 93% good or excellent clinical results with follow-up of up to 33 years. The failures were early, caused by infection and oversizing of the implant. In the study by Townley and Taranow,[37] the preoperative diagnoses included hallux valgus, rheumatoid arthritis, and hallux rigidus; however, most failures (11 of 13) occurred in patients with hallux valgus and rheumatoid arthritis. This study demonstrated encouraging long-term results for patients with hallux rigidus using this hemiarthroplasty prosthesis. In addition, because of the inert material of the implant and minimal bone resection required for the operation, the longevity of this procedure avoided the pitfalls identified in other arthroplasty designs. **Fig. 4** shows the Townley implant inserted into the proximal phalanx of the great toe. A cheilectomy of the joint has been performed at the same time.

There remain limitations to the application of Townley's data for patients with severe hallux rigidus. The study lacked a prospective collection of data and there is limited objective information for patient selection and outcomes. It does not have the problems associated with silicone and is not difficult to revise to an arthrodesis.

The techniques of resurfacing the MTP joint[38] involve a dorsal cheilectomy of the first metatarsal and the proximal phalanx. Postoperatively, early range of motion is encouraged and the patients can fully weight bear. The metatarsosesamoid articulation can cause pain in the joint just as the patellofemoral joint can in knee arthroplasty. This is relevant for procedures that increase the total range of motion in the joint and increase motion in the sesamoid-metatarsal articulation.

Beeson and colleagues[7] highlight the need for a prospective study to develop a suitable classification system for the condition. The role of the sesamoids and the effect of arthritis of the metatarsosesamoid joint cannot be underestimated particularly in evaluating treatment options. Arthritis surgery of the knee takes into consideration the patellofemoral joint and when considering the best treatment option for arthritis

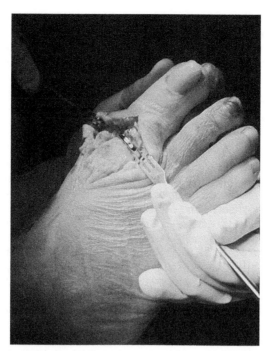

Fig. 4. The Townley implant after it has been inserted into the proximal phalanx of the great toe.

in the great toe, the sesamoid-metatarsal joint cannot be ignored. **Fig. 5** depicts the CT scans of arthritis involving the metatarsosesamoid articulation in the first MTP joint.

Resection of the sesamoid osteophytes at the time of the hemiarthroplasty has been described and although it is possible to do, it is likely to be unpredictable in leading to relief of pain when the sesamoid arthritis is extensive and severe. More research needs to be done on the preoperative grading of hallux rigidus using CT scanning and the role of sesamoid arthritis in the poor outcomes following hemiarthroplasty.

Taranow and coworkers[39] reviewed 28 patients who underwent hemiarthroplasty with an average follow-up of 33 months. A total of 5 out of 28 patients were not completely satisfied with the procedure. Four patients had implants inserted in

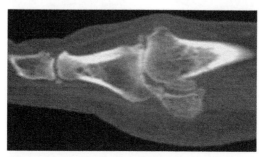

Fig. 5. CT scan of metatarsosesamoid arthritis with large osteophytes inferiorly on the proximal phalanx, metatarsal head, and the sesamoids.

a dorsiflexed position with the stem impinging against the plantar cortex of the proximal phalanx. Three implants showed evidence of subsidence and loosening, which the authors attribute to technical errors. Taranow believes the simplicity of the design and use of a durable material eliminates the risk of mechanical failure of the implant. The implant does allow minimal bone resection, although their recommendation of resecting more bone than the width of the implant is questionable because this increases the risk of shortening the toe and of transfer metatarsalgia developing. The importance of not resecting more than the 2 mm width of the implant from the proximal phalanx has been recently highlighted,[38] because further shortening of the great toe can lead to the problems of transfer metatarsalgia.

Fig. 6 illustrates the technique of using the instrumentation to determine the width of bone resection on the proximal phalanx, which is equal to the width of the implant. Using either the small or small-medium implant is important because the larger implants can lead to stiffness and overstuffing the joint.

Jelinek and coworkers[40] presented a retrospective study on 41 toes over a 6-year period. There were seven revisions (17%) with an average of 29 months to revision. The satisfaction rate was 67%. Their results did not match those of Townley.

Raikin and coworkers[41] compared the Townley hemiarthroplasty with an arthrodesis of the first MTP joint. This was a retrospective case control study. Eight of the hemiarthroplasties that were not considered failures had radiographic cutout of the distal portion of the implant through the plantar cortex of the proximal phalanx. This raises some concern regarding the technique used for the hemiarthroplasty. They reported a higher incidence of long-term failure with the Townley hemiarthroplasty but emphasized that the procedure requires minimal bone resection thereby

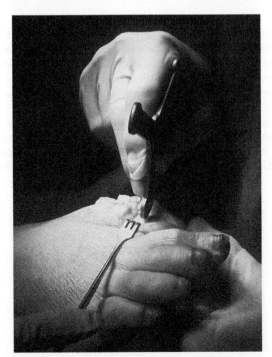

Fig. 6. The template is used to mark the line of resection of the proximal phalanx. The width of this equals the width of the implant.

facilitating conversion to an arthrodesis if required without great difficulty or structural bone graft. They concluded that arthrodesis was more predictable than hemiarthroplasty in alleviating symptoms and restoring function.

The results of 21 Townley hemiarthroplasties were presented by Aronow and coworkers.[42] The authors believe the least satisfied patients had less aggressive dorsal cheilectomies at the time of implant insertion. Prosthesis subsidence and surrounding radiolucency did not seem to correlate with patient dissatisfaction. They concluded that the procedure remained a viable option for grade 3 hallux rigidus.

Sorbie and Saunders[43] recently published results using the Trihedron cobalt chrome cemented hemiarthroplasty technique. A total of 19 patients were in the study and the follow-up was 34 to 72 months on 23 cases. They believe the implant to be safe and effective in the short term in the treatment of hallux rigidus. There was no evidence of loosening of the components at an average of 5-year follow-up. All patients had increased range of motion postoperatively.

The indications for hemiarthroplasty remain to be defined. Hemiarthroplasty may be seen as an alternative to arthrodesis in some cases. It can be an additional option for some patients who do not benefit from a cheilectomy and for whom the arthrodesis has possible functional limitations. To date the evidence supporting the use of hemiarthroplasty is of poor quality and conflicting.[44]

Resurfacing of the metatarsal was introduced in 2005 with Arthrosurface HemiCAP. This system is supposed to provide reconstruction of an anatomic joint surface by using a series of articular components made up of a cobalt-chrome alloy for the articular portion attached to a titanium alloy taper post. The initial use of this device was in other joints, such as the knee. Hasselman and Shields[45] described the results of more than 100 patients using the HemiCAP. There were two failures, one from infection and one from metallosis. The mean follow-up was 20 months. There was a mean postoperative increase in range of motion of 42 degrees. They state that 25 of the first 30 patients were stage 2 or stage 3 hallux rigidus. There were no reports of implant loosening or osteolysis. The authors believe that the screw fixation component may provide a stronger construct and be less likely to loosen. There is no mention of the ease or difficulty of revising this prosthesis if it fails.

One study reported on 24 HemiCAP procedures with an average duration follow-up of 12 months. The average AOFAS score improved from 54 to 70 postoperatively and average dorsiflexion increased 30 degrees. There are no long-term data on the effectiveness of this device for the treatment of hallux rigidus.

TOTAL TOE ARTHROPLASTY

Metal-on-polyethylene total toe implants are available and consist of porous coated titanium stems inserted in a press fit or cemented fashion. They have a cobalt-chrome articulating surface with polyethylene. The Biomet design has a sesamoid articulation on the plantar condylar surface of the metatarsal head component. Koenig and Horwitz[46] published results of 61 patients with this prosthesis; however, the indications were varied in this group of patients including a group who were having salvage of a failed Silastic implant. Understandably, these patients fared poorly.

Fuhrmann and coworkers[47] published the results of a modular, nonconstrained, porous-coated prosthesis known as the "Reflexion" prosthesis. The average follow-up period was 3 years. Because of poor bone quality they cemented-in almost half of the phalangeal components. Despite this a significant amount of patients developed instability in both the axial and sagittal planes. Radiolucency around 23% of the phalangeal components and 10% of the metatarsal components was reported.

Ess and coworkers[48] had 10 patients with hallux rigidus treated with the Reflexion prosthesis. At the 2-year follow-up, four were rated as fair or poor. Malalignment occurred in three of the implants and one component was loose. They recommended not using the implant in active people.

Konkel and Menger[49] published short-term results of the Swanson titanium great toe implant. The 12 patients were classified as grade 2 or grade 3 hallux rigidus, although the grading system is not mentioned. The authors mention debriding osteophytes on the sesamoid as part of the operative technique; however, the extent of sesamoid-metatarsal arthritis in the first MTP joint in their group of patients is not mentioned. A cheilectomy was performed at the same time as insertion of the implant into the proximal phalanx. They recommend in their operative technique resecting 1 to 2 mm more of the base of the proximal phalanx than required for the titanium implant, which leads to overall shortening of the great toe. The risk is this could lead to transfer metatarsalgia and they report one of the patients requiring a Weil osteotomy of the metatarsal. Although they reported satisfactory results in 10 of the 12 patients, all patients developed radiolucencies and subsidence of the implant.

Pulavarti and coworkers[50] reviewed 36 patients with a minimum follow-up of 3 years using the Bio-Action prosthesis. This is a nonconstrained uncemented implant. A total of 78% of patients rated the implant as excellent or good. Two patients required salvage surgery and one third of the group had radiographic evidence of loosening and subsidence.

Gibson and Thomson[51] compared arthrodesis of the first MTP joint and total replacement arthroplasty in patients with symptomatic hallux rigidus. This was a prospective randomized controlled study. At 2-year follow-up, the arthrodesis group (38 feet) reported 82% improvement compared with 45% after arthroplasty (39 feet). Loosening of the phalangeal component was found in six patients. A total of 40% of patients would not undergo the total replacement arthroplasty again. They concluded that arthrodesis was superior to total joint replacement.

Overall, the reported complication rate of total toe implants is considerable. It is difficult at the moment to recommend the use of total toe implants when one compares it with the results of other treatment modalities.

REFERENCES

1. Defrino PF, Brodsky JW, Pollo FE, et al. First metatarsophalangeal arthrodesis: a clinical, pedobarographic and gait analysis study. Foot Ankle Int 2002;23: 496–502.
2. Giannini S, Ceccarelli F, Faldini C, et al. What's new in surgical options for hallux rigidus? J Bone Joint Surg Am 2004;86-A(Suppl 2):72–83.
3. Shereff MJ, Baumhauer JF. Hallux rigidus and osteoarthrosis of the first metatarsophalangeal joint. J Bone Joint Surg Am 1998;80:898–908.
4. VanGheluwe BR, Dananberg HJ, Hagman F, et al. Effects of hallux limitus on plantar foot pressure and kinematics during walking. J Am Podiatr Med Assoc 2006;96:428–36.
5. Nawoczenski DA, Ketz J, Baumhauer J. Dynamic kinematic and plantar pressure changes following cheilectomy for hallux rigidus: a mid-term follow up. Foot Ankle Int 2008;29:265–72.
6. Easley M, Davis WH, Anderson RB. Intermediate to long term follow up of medial - approach dorsal cheilectomy for hallux rigidus. Foot Ankle Int 1999;20(3):147–52.
7. Beeson P, Phillips C, Corr S, et al. Classification systems for hallux rigidus: a review of the literature. Foot Ankle Int 2008;29(4):407–14.

8. Coughlin MJ, Shurnas PS. Hallux rigidus: grading and long term results of operative treatment. J Bone Joint Surg Am 2003;85A:2072–88.
9. Citron N, Neil M. Dorsal wedge osteotomy of the proximal phalanx for hallux rigidus: long term results. J Bone Joint Surg Br 1987;69:835–7.
10. Coughlin MJ. Arthrodesis of the first metatarsophalangeal joint. Orthop Rev 1990; 19:177–86.
11. Coughlin MJ. Arthrodesis of the first metatarsophalangeal joint with mini-fragment plate fixation. Orthopaedics 1990;13:1037–44.
12. Coughlin MJ, Abdo RV. Arthrodesis of the first metatarsophalangeal joint with Vitallium plate fixation. Foot Ankle Int 1994;15:18–28.
13. Coughlin MJ, Grebing BR, Jones CP. Arthrodesis of the first metatarsophalangeal joint for idiopathic hallux valgus: intermediate results. Foot Ankle Int 2005;26:783–92.
14. Fitzgerald JAW. A review of the long term results of arthrodesis of the first metatarsophalangeal joint. J Bone Joint Surg 1969;51-B:488–93.
15. Mann RA, Oates JC. Arthrodesis of the first metatarsophalangeal joint. Foot Ankle Int 1980;1:159–66.
16. Turan I, Lindgren U. Compression-screw arthrodesis of the first metatarsophalangeal joint of the foot. Clin Orthop 1987;221:292–5.
17. Goucher NR, Coughlin MJ. Hallux metatarsophalangeal joint arthrodesis using dome shaped reamers and dorsal plate fixation: a prospective study. Foot Ankle Int 2006;27(11):869–76.
18. Esway J, Conti S. Joint replacement in the hallux metatarsophalangeal joint. Foot Ankle Clin 2005;10:97–115.
19. Wenger RJ, Whalley RC. Total replacement of the first metatarsophalangeal joint. J Bone Joint Surg 1978;60B(1):88–92.
20. Cracchiolo A, Weltmer JB, Lian G, et al. Arthroplasty of the first metatarsophalangeal joint with a double stem silicone implant: results in patients who have degenerative joint disease failure of previous operations or rheumatoid arthritis. J Bone Joint Surg Am 1992;74A(4):552–63.
21. Swanson AB, Swanson GD, Manpin K, et al. The use of a grommet bone liner for flexible hinge implant arthroplasty of the great toe. Foot Ankle 1991;12(3):149–55.
22. Swanson AB, Swanson GD. Use of grommets for flexible hinge implant arthroplasty of the great toe. Clin Orthop 1997;340:87–94.
23. Granberry WM, Noble PC, Bishop JO, et al. Use of a hinged silicone prosthesis for replacement of the first metatarsophalangeal joint. J Bone Joint Surg 1991; 73-A:1453–9.
24. Hecht PJ, Gibbons MJ, Wapner KL, et al. Arthrodesis of the first metatarsophalangeal joint to salvage failed silicone arthroplasty. Foot Ankle Int 1997;18(7):383–90.
25. Kitaoka HB, Holiday AD, Chao EY, et al. Salvage of failed first metatarsophalangeal joint implant arthroplasty by implant removal and synovectomy: clinical and biomechanical evaluation. Foot Ankle Int 1992;13(5):243–50.
26. Brewood AFM, Griffiths JC. The long term results of silicone stem Silastic arthroplasty of the great toe. J R Coll Surg Edinb 1985;30:159–61.
27. Shankar NS. Silastic single stem implants in the treatment of hallux rigidus. Foot Ankle Int 1995;16(8):487–91.
28. Shankar NS, Assad SS, Craxford AD. Hinged Silastic implants of the great toe. Clin Orthop 1991;272:227–34.
29. Verhaar J, Vermeulen A, Bulstra S, et al. Bone reaction to silicone metatarsophalangeal joint hemiprosthesis. Clin Orthop 1989;245:228–32.
30. Shereff MJ, Jahss MH. Complications of Silastic implant arthroplasty in the hallux. Foot Ankle 1980;1:95–101.

31. Johnson KA, Saltzman CL. Complications of resection arthroplasty and replacement arthroplasty procedures. Contemp Orthop 1991;23:139–47.
32. Lemon RA, Engber WD, McBeath AA. A complication of Silastic hemiarthroplasty in bunion surgery. Foot Ankle Int 1984;4:262–6.
33. Rahman H, Fagg PS. Silicone granulomatous reactions after first metatarsophalangeal hemiarthroplasty. J Bone Joint Surg Br 1993;75 B(4):637–9.
34. Freed JB. The increasing recognition of medullary lysis, cortical osteophytic proliferation, and fragmentation of implanted silicone polymer implants. J Foot Ankle Surg 1993;32(2):171–9.
35. McNearney T, Haque A, Wen J, et al. Inguinal lymph node foreign body granulomas after placement of a silicone implant of the first metatarsophalangeal joint. J Rheumatol 1996;23(8):1449–52.
36. Sammarco GJ, Tbatowski K. Silicone lymphadenopathy associated with failed prosthesis of the hallux: a case report and literature review. Foot Ankle 1992; 13(5):273–6.
37. Townley CO, Taranow WS. A metallic hemiarthroplasty resurfacing prosthesis for the hallux metatarsophalangeal joint. Foot Ankle Int 1994;15(11):575–80.
38. Giza E, Sullivan MR. First metatarsophalangeal hemiarthroplasty for grade 3 and 4 hallux rigidus. Tech Foot Ankle Surg 2005;4:2–9.
39. Taranow WS, Moutsatson MJ, Cooper JM. Contemporary approaches to stage 2 and 3 hallux rigidus: the role of metallic hemiarthroplasty of the proximal phalanx. Foot Ankle Clin 2005;10:713–28.
40. Jellinek A, Anderson J, Bohay D. Management of hallux rigidus: the metallic hemiarthroplasty resurfacing prosthesis revisited. AOFAS 23rd Annual Summer Meeting. La Jolla, CA, July 14–16, 2006.
41. Raikin S, Ahmad J, Pour A, et al. A comparison of arthrodesis and the BioPro Metallic Hemiarthroplasty of the hallux metatarsophalangeal joint. AOFAS 23rd Annual Summer Meeting. La Jolla, CA, July 14–16, 2006.
42. Aronow M, Leger R, Sullivan R. The results of first MTP joint hemiarthroplasty in grade 3 hallux rigidus. AOFAS 23rd Annual Summer Meeting. La Jolla, CA, July 14–16, 2006.
43. Sorbie C, Saunders GA. Hemiarthroplasty in the treatment of hallux rigidus. Foot Ankle Int 2008;29(3):273–81.
44. Yee G, Lau J. Current concepts review: hallux rigidus. Foot Ankle Int 2008;29(6): 637–46.
45. Hasselman C, Shields N. Resurfacing of the first metatarsal head in the treatment of hallux rigidus. Tech Foot Ankle Surg 2008;7(1):31–40.
46. Koenig RD, Horwitz LR. The Biomet total toe system utilizing the Koenig score: a five year review. J Foot Ankle Surg 1996;35(1):23–6.
47. Fuhrmann RA, Wagner A, Anders JO. First metatarsophalangeal joint replacement: the method of choice for end stage hallux rigidus? Foot Ankle Clin 2003;8:711–21.
48. Ess P, Hamalainen M, Leppilkahti J. Non-constrained titanium-polyethylene total endoprosthesis in the treatment of hallux rigidus. Scand J Surg 2002;91:202–7.
49. Konkel KF, Menger AG. Mid-term results of titanium hemi-great toe implants. Foot Ankle Int 2006;27(11):922–9.
50. Pulvarti RS, McVie JL, Tulloch CJ. First metatarsophalangeal joint replacement using the bio-action great toe implant: intermediate results. Foot Ankle Int 2005;26(12):1033–7.
51. Gibson A, Thomson CE. Arthrodesis or total replacement arthroplasty for hallux rigidus. Foot Ankle Int 2005;26(9):680–90.

First Metatarsophalangeal Arthrodesis

John W. Womack, MD[a], Susan N. Ishikawa, MD[b],*

KEYWORDS

- Metatarsophalangeal arthrodesis • Implant arthroplasty
- Hallux rigidus • Arthritis • Fusion • Hallux
- Metatarsophalangeal joint • Cup and cone reamers

Arthrodesis of the first metatarsophalangeal (MTP) joint is a highly successful treatment for patients with symptomatic hallux rigidus who have failed conservative management. The primary indications for hallux MTP fusion are severe hallux rigidus or as a salvage procedure for failed cheilectomy, resection arthroplasty, or implant arthroplasty. Additionally, MTP arthrodesis is appropriate for severe hallux valgus or hallux varus deformities with concomitant arthritis. Before arthrodesis, the importance of host factors, such as use of nicotine, local blood supply, medical comorbidites, and use of systemic immunosuppressive agents, must be considered.[1] Reported fusion rates after arthrodesis range from 90% to 100% in the literature.[2] When nonunion occurs it may be fibrous and painless.[2] Arthrodesis is currently considered the gold standard treatment for end-stage arthritis of the MTP joint. Careful attention to surgical detail is critical to achieving optimal outcomes.

SURGICAL CONSIDERATIONS
Biomechanical Considerations

Although the main objective for MTP arthrodesis is pain relief and restoration of function, sacrificing the motion of the first MTP joint has biomechanical consequences, both positive and negative. DeFrino and colleagues[3] show that fusing a painful joint allows greater weightbearing of the hallux postoperatively, but there are subtle gait changes to compensate for the loss of first MTP motion, which include loss in ankle plantarflexion moment and ankle power at toe-off. Studies have shown, however, that eliminating motion at the first MTP joint does not cause any observable change in the gait patterns of those patients who have undergone the procedure.[4]

[a] Piedmont Orthopaedic Associates, 35 International Drive, Greenville, SC 29615, USA
[b] University of Tennessee/Campbell Clinic, 1458 West Poplar Avenue, Suite 100, Collierville, TN 38017, USA
* Corresponding author.
E-mail address: sishikawa@campbellclinic.com (S.N. Ishikawa).

Foot Ankle Clin N Am 14 (2009) 43–50
doi:10.1016/j.fcl.2008.11.008
1083-7515/08/$ – see front matter © 2009 Elsevier Inc. All rights reserved.

foot.theclinics.com

Fixation Options

Many fixation techniques ranging from Kirschner wires, staples, external fixation, plates and screws, and crossed screws have been used with success.[1] Many studies have examined the biomechanics of various internal fixation techniques because external fixation is rarely used. The use of chromic catgut in one British series demonstrated a 90% union rate[5] and intraosseus wiring has shown a 56% to 96% rate of union.[6] Contemporary literature focuses on rigid internal fixation with screws and plates. Rongstad and colleagues[7] compared the fixation strength of a single, oblique 4-mm cancellous screw with a 4.5-mm Herbert screw, a 3/32 threaded axial pin, and a dorsal Vitallium plate. The dorsal plate and Herbert screw construct were the strongest. The single 4-mm screw and the Steinmann pin were comparable in strength. A headless variable compression screw has also been used and may help prevent painful hardware and dorsal cortical breakout from impingement of the head of the screw on the metatarsal shaft.[8] Watson and Kelkian[9] have also examined the cost effectiveness of various implants. They compared a variable headless compression screw (Herbert), small fragment screws, and a dorsal compression plate. The small fragment screws were found to have the lowest average cost of use when union rate and cost of fixation systems were taken into account.

The method of preparing the fusion site has also been studied, demonstrating that a cup-and-cone configuration is biomechanically more sound than flat bone cuts.[10] Goucher and Coughlin[11] have shown that the use of a commercially available cup and cone reamer system has great ease of use and leads to predictable outcomes. They report a 92% union rate using a cup and cone reamer technique and a precontoured dorsal titanium plate, with no hardware failures. They argue that although flat cuts may be simple to make, any change that must be made affects two other planes and further shortens the first ray. A cup and cone system allows the surgeon to "dial in" the desired valgus, dorsiflexion, and rotation with infinite variability. This technique does, however, require a more extensive exposure to allow the reamer to be aligned directly down the shafts of the metatarsal and proximal phalanx.

ARTHRODESIS POSITIONING

The alignment of the great toe is perhaps the most critical of all the technical considerations in MTP arthrodesis. Although authors have shown that fibrous nonunions can be quite forgiving,[2] the same cannot be said about a malpositioned hallux. Kelikian[1] notes that one of the pitfalls in arthrodesis positioning is reliance on the first metatarsal declination angle for the reference point of the hallux. Because of variations in the foot, such as metatarsus elevatus, cavus, or pes planus, he argues that the floor or flat weight-bearing surface is the best reference point on which to base the alignment of the hallux in the sagittal plane. Dorsiflexion of the hallux from 10 to 40 degrees has been advocated in the literature.[12,13] Because the first metatarsal declination angle can vary between 15 and 30 degrees, it is preferable to use the position of the phalanx relative to the floor as a reference point.[1] The ideal dorsiflexion is between 10 and 15 degrees. Excessive dorsiflexion is not well tolerated because of dorsal irritation of the interphalangeal joint with shoewear. The most effective method of intraoperative assessment of the dorsiflexion of the hallux is the use of a flat sterile instrument tray with the ankle held in neutral dorsiflexion to simulate weight bearing. The great toe should be in 10 to 15 degrees of dorsiflexion relative to the tray.[12,13] Alexander[14] points out that if the tip of the toe clears the box top by 4 to 8 mm, then the position of the hallux is optimal to allow normal toe-off with limited risk of hallux overload. Some authors advocate increasing the dorsiflexion to 15 degrees of extension in women to allow the wearing of a low heel.[1,15] This recommendation should be approached with caution, however, because excessive dorsiflexion in shoes other than heels can lead to interphalangeal joint irritation in these patients. Use of an Esmarch tourniquet around the ankle can also increase tension on the extensor hallucis longus (EHL) tendon and affect the position of the phalanx when trying to evaluate positioning of the arthrodesis in the sagittal plane. If an Esmarch is used in this fashion, it is important to take this factor into consideration before provisional fixation of the arthrodesis.

Frontal plane alignment should be between 10 and 15 degrees of valgus. Varus positioning causes impingement of the toe against the inner surface of the shoe toe-box and has also been demonstrated to accelerate interphalangeal joint arthritis, whereas excessive valgus leads to impingement against the second toe.[16] Axial plane alignment is rarely a problem when MTP arthrodesis is performed for hallux rigidus. Rotational alignment is best evaluated by referencing the position of the nail bed relative to the lesser toes.

SURGICAL TECHNIQUE
Exposure

A dorsal incision is made down to the capsule and the EHL tendon is identified. A capsulotomy is made just lateral to the EHL tendon, leaving a 2- to 3-mm cuff of capsule left to repair at closure. A rongeur is used to debride osteophytes and chronic synovitis in and around the first MTP joint. A wide Hohmann retractor is placed on the lateral side of the metatarsal head to retract the soft tissues throughout the remainder of the procedure. Commercially available conical reamers can then be used to remove the articular cartilage from the metatarsal head and the base of the proximal phalanx (**Fig. 1**). This usually requires dislocation of the first MTP joint so that the guidewire can be placed directly down the shaft on either side of the joint. Both arthrodesis surfaces are sequentially reamed until all of the subchondral bone has been removed and bleeding cancellous bone is exposed. Care must be taken in osteoporotic bone to avoid overreaming and shortening of the bone surfaces.

Alternatively, a medial incision may also be used and may be more cosmetically appealing. A medial incision may make circumferential exposure of the joint more difficult, however, and can risk injury to the dorsomedial cutaneous nerve of the hallux. If a medial incision is used, a longitudinal arthrotomy is created by elevating dorsal and plantar flaps. Flat saw cuts are then made with a sagittal saw but they must be precise to allow proper positioning of the arthrodesis site. It is necessary to avoid excessive shortening of the bones while creating these saw cuts. One technique tip that has

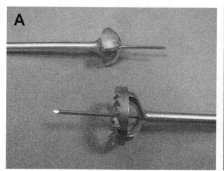 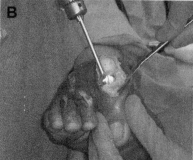

Fig. 1. (*A, B*) Cup and cone reamers.

been reported is the use of a crescentic blade to make appropriate cuts on the meta-tarsal and the proximal phalanx.[17] At this point, a Kirschner wire can be used to drill holes into the cancellous bone to create vascular channels and allow for increased blood flow at the arthrodesis site.

Regardless of the method of joint preparation, the arthrodesis site is then reduced into the desired position and alignment is checked in all three planes. Fluoroscopic evaluation and clinical assessment with use of a sterile flat surface, such as the cover of an instrument tray, can greatly assist in ensuring appropriate positioning. Once satisfactory alignment has been confirmed, the arthrodesis site is provisionally fixed with Kirschner wires or guide pins from a cannulated screw system.

Fixation

The use of a cannulated screw system for fixation allows more accurate placement of hardware and the ability to confirm position with fluoroscopy before drilling through the arthrodesis site. The use of headless compression screws offers an attractive option to small fragment screws because less hardware irritation occurs with this fixation method. Crossed screws are commonly used with one screw placed from distal-medial to proximal-lateral and one screw placed from proximal-medial to distal-lateral (**Fig. 2**). It should be noted that screw fixation can create stress risers in the arthrodesis site and periprosthetic fractures can be a concern. A 3-mm burr can be used to smooth the dorsal lip of the screw hole to relieve stress on the bone interface by creating a gliding hole before final screw insertion.

In cases of severe osteopenia, inadequate screw fixation strength, or revision procedures, dorsal compression plating presents a viable supplement. Many commercially available precontoured plates are available on the market today. These plates typically have 10 degrees of valgus angulation and 9 degrees of extension. It should be noted that occasional contouring of the plate is required with plate benders if the plate contour does not match the desired position of the arthrodesis. Screw

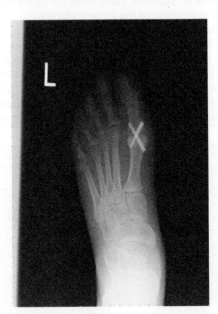

Fig. 2. MTP arthrodesis with crossed headless compressions screws.

placement in compression should begin with a neutral screw in the phalanx and proceed proximally in the plate. Screw depth should be measured carefully to avoid injury to the sesamoid complex. Use of the plate can be supplemented with a lag screw placed directly across the arthrodesis site (**Fig. 3**).

Postoperative Treatment

The capsule is closed using a 2-0 absorbable suture and the skin is closed using 4-0 nylon suture. A compressive forefoot bandage is applied, followed by a well-padded posterior splint. The sutures are removed at 2 weeks postoperatively. Touch down weight bearing with crutches and a prefabricated walking boot can be initiated at that time if the fixation seems solid intraoperatively. A radiograph is obtained at 4 weeks postoperatively and progression to full weight bearing is allowed if the arthrodesis seems stable. Transition into postoperative hard-soled shoe and then into normal shoe wear typically occurs between weeks 6 and 10. Return to high-impact activities is allowed at 16 weeks if the radiograph seems satisfactory.

Clinical Outcomes of Hallux Metatarsophalangeal Arthrodesis for Hallux Rigidus

First MTP arthrodesis has been shown to have good outcomes in numerous studies. Fusion rates with appropriate fixation have been 90% to 100% and patient satisfaction has been uniformly high.[18] Some of the more recent studies include one by Coughlin and Shurnas,[2] who have demonstrated a 94% fusion rate and good or excellent subjective results in 100% of patients with an average 6.7-years follow-up in patients with advanced hallux rigidus. Brodsky and colleagues[19] had a 100% fusion rate in 60 feet at an average follow-up of 44 months. There was a 94% patient satisfaction rate and most patients went back to former sporting activities including running, tennis, and golf. Goucher and Coughlin[11] reported on 49 patients who had undergone first MTP arthrodesis for numerous diagnoses with a minimum 1-year follow-up. There was a 92% fusion rate and 96% satisfaction rate with a significant improvement in pain scores and American Orthopaedic Foot and Ankle Society (AOFAS) scores. Of the four nonunions, three rated themselves as having a good result; the fourth had a fair result. Flavin and Stephens[20] reported on 12 patients with a variety of diagnoses, with an average 18-month follow-up. There was a 100% fusion rate and improvement in AOFAS scores and short form-36 (SF-36) scores.

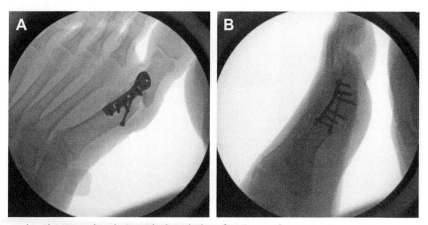

Fig. 3. (A, B) MTP arthrodesis with dorsal plate fixation and compression screw.

COMPARISON OF METATARSOPHALANGEAL ARTHRODESIS WITH IMPLANT ARTHROPLASTY FOR HALLUX RIGIDUS

Although joint replacement remains the ultimate solution for hip and knee arthritis, and may be a viable option in ankle arthritis, implant arthroplasty of the hallux MTP joint has not yet been demonstrated to be superior to fusion for treating hallux rigidus. MTP arthrodesis remains the gold standard for surgical treatment of the severely arthritic MTP joint.[1,21–23] Numerous types of MTP implants have been developed since the 1970s. The first implants were metals and acrylics. Early failures of these implants led to the advent of Silastic single-stem and double-stem implants. Complications with Silastic implants emerged in the 1980s, including devastating osteolysis, late failures, foreign body immune response, and fracture of the implants. The first metal-on-polyethylene implant was introduced in 1990. Numerous prostheses have attained Food and Drug Administration class II approval through the less stringent 510(k) process. Currently, there are three Silastic double-stemmed hinges, four metal hemi-arthroplasty implants, and four metal-on-polyethylene products available on the market (**Fig. 4**).[15]

Numerous retrospective (level IV) series in the literature discuss outcomes of first MTP implant arthroplasty with short- to mid-term follow-up. There are higher-quality studies, however, directly comparing implant arthroplasty with arthrodesis for hallux rigidus. Gibson and Thompson[24] published a noteworthy randomized controlled (level I) trial evaluating clinical outcomes after first MTP arthrodesis versus replacement arthroplasty for late-stage hallux rigidus. Between 1998 and 2001, 63 patients were randomized to fusion (38 toes) or replacement arthroplasty (39 toes). All procedures were performed by a single surgeon and pain was assessed with a visual analog scale measured at 6 months, 12 months, and 2 years postoperatively. Both groups showed pain improvement at 24 months, but six of the implants in the arthroplasty group had to be removed because of component loosening and gross failure. The implant arthroplasty patients had a poor range of motion and dynamic pedobarograph

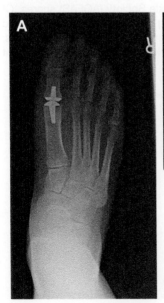
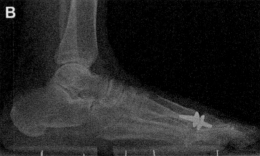

Fig. 4. (*A, B*) MTP arthroplasty.

study indicated increased pressures on the lateral border of the foot. The authors concluded that even if the data from the early implant failures were excluded, patients clearly preferred arthrodesis over implant arthroplasty.

Raikin and colleagues[25] reported a retrospective comparative (level III) study evaluating arthrodesis versus implant hemiarthroplasty. They compared the outcomes of arthrodesis of the MTP joint performed by a single surgeon with implant arthroplasties performed by a second surgeon. Patients were evaluated by an independent observer using the AOFAS Hallux Metatarsophalangeal Interphalangeal scoring system. Seventeen patients who underwent hemiarthroplasty were available for review with a mean follow-up of 79.2 months. Five (24%) of these patients required additional surgery at an average of 13 months after the index procedure because of hemiarthroplasty failure. Eight of the patients in which the prosthesis had survived showed radiographic evidence of plantar cutout on the final follow-up radiograph. All 27 arthrodesis patients achieved union and no revisions were required. The mean AOFAS score at final follow-up was significantly higher in the arthrodesis group. They concluded that MTP arthrodesis offers a more predictable outcome than hemiarthroplasty for hallux rigidus, with a lower complication rate and a higher long-term satisfaction rate.

Although a major advantage of implant arthroplasty over arthrodesis is the theoretic preservation of MTP range of motion, the literature to support this claim is sparse. Only two studies directly assessed postoperative range of motion of implant arthroplasties. Ashford and colleagues,[26] in the podiatric literature, showed average dorsiflexion of patients undergoing Silastic double-stemmed arthroplasty to be 21 degrees (range, 6–46 degrees), whereas Gibson and Thompson[24] reported range of motion as poor even in patients who had not had an implant failure.

Raikin and colleagues[25] conclude that because of the high rate of early implant failure and evidence of radiographic loosening in many patients, arthrodesis remains superior to implant arthroplasty for treatment of symptomatic late-grade hallux rigidus. As they point out, a recent publication by Brodsky and colleagues on long-term follow-up of first MTP arthrodesis showed a 94% satisfaction rate, a 100% union rate, and effective pain relief. The authors are not aware of any results in the arthroplasty literature that can approach these results.

REFERENCES

1. Kelikian AS. Technical considerations in hallux metarsophalangeal arthodesis. Foot Ankle Clin 2005;10:167–90.
2. Coughlin MJ, Shurnas PS. Hallux rigidus: grading and long-term results of operative treatment. J Bone Joint Surg Am 2003;85-A(11):2072–88.
3. DeFrino PF, Brodsky JW, Pollo F, et al. First metatarsophalangeal arthrodesis: a clinical, pedobarographic and gait analysis study. Foot Ankle Int 2002;23(6): 496–502.
4. Mann RA, Oates JC. Arthrodesis of the first metatarsophalangeal joint. Foot Ankle 1980;1(3):159–66.
5. Chana GS, Andrew TA, Cotterill CP. A simple method of arthrodesis of the first metatarsophalangeal joint. J Bone Joint Surg Br 1984;66:703–5.
6. O'Doherty DP, Lowrie IG, Magnussen PA, et al. The management of the painful first metatarsophalangeal joint in the older patient: arthrodesis or Keller's arthroplasty? J Bone Joint Surg Br 1990;72(5):839–42.
7. Rongstad DJ, Miller GJ, Vadergriend RA, et al. A biomechanical comparison of four fixation methods of first metatarsophalangeal joint arthrodesis. Foot Ankle Int 1994;15:415–9.

8. Wu KK. Fusion of the metatarsophalangeal joint of the great toe with Herbert screws. Foot Ankle 1993;14:165–9.

9. Watson AD, Kelkian AS. Cost-effectiveness comparison of three methods of internal fixation for arthrodesis of the first metatarsophalangeal joint. Foot Ankle Int 1998;19:304–10.

10. Curtis MJ, Myerson M, Jinnah RH, et al. Arthrodesis of the first metatarsophalangeal joint: a biomechanical study of internal fixation techniques. Foot Ankle Int 1993;14:395–9.

11. Goucher NR, Coughlin MJ. Hallux metatarsophalangeal joint arthrodesis using dome-shaped reamers and dorsal plate fixation: a prospective study. Foot Ankle Int 2006;27:869–76.

12. Harper MC. Positioning of the hallux for first metatarsophalangeal joint arthrodesis. Foot Ankle Int 1997;18:827.

13. Conti SF, Dhawan S. Arthrodesis of the first metatarsophalageal and interphalangeal joints of the foot. Foot Ankle Clin 1996;1:33–53.

14. Alexander IJ. Hallux metartarsophalangeal joint arthrodesis. In: Kitakoa HB, editor. Masters techniques in foot and ankle surgery. 2nd edition. Philadelphia: Lippincott Williams and Wilkins; 2002. p. 45–60.

15. Esway JE, Conti SF. Joint replacement in the hallux metatarsophalangeal joint. Foot Ankle Clin 2005;10(10):97–115.

16. Fitzgerald JAW. A review of long-term results of first metatarsophalangeal arthrodesis. J Bone Joint Surg Br 1969;51:488–93.

17. Shute GC, Sferra JJ. Use of the crescentic saw for arthrodesis of the first metatarsophalangeal joint. Foot Ankle Int 1998;19(100):719–20.

18. Yee G, Lau J. Current concepts review: hallux rigidus. Foot Ankle Int 2008;29(6):637–46.

19. Brodsky JW, Passmore RN, Pollo FE, et al. Functional outcome of arthrodesis of the first metatarsophalangeal joint using parallel screw fixation. Foot Ankle Int 2005;26:140–6.

20. Flavin R, Stephens MM. Arthrodesis of the first metatarsophalangeal joint using a dorsal titanium contoured plate. Foot Ankle Int 2004;25(11):783–7.

21. Weinfeld SB, Schon LC. Hallux metatarsophalangeal arthritis. Clin Orthop Relat Res 1998;349:9–19.

22. Giannini S, Ceccarelli F, Faldini C, et al. What's new in surgical options for hallux rigidus? J Bone Joint Surg Am 2004;86-A(Suppl 2):72–83.

23. Sammarco VJ, Nichols R. Orthotic management for disorders of the hallux. Foot Ankle Clin 2005;10(1):191–209.

24. Gibson J, Thomson CE. Arthrodesis or total replacement surgery for hallux rigidus: a randomized controlled trial. Foot Ankle Int 2005;26(9):680–90.

25. Raikin SM, Ahmad J, Pour AE, et al. Comparison of arthrodesis and metallic hemiarthroplasty of the hallux metatarsophalangeal joint. J Bone Joint Surg Am 2007;89(9):1979–85.

26. Ashford RL, Vogiatozoglou Tollafield DR, Casella JP. Retrospective analysis of Swanson Silastic double-stemmed great toe implants with titanium grommets following podiatric surgery for arthritic joint disease. The Foot 2000;10:69–74.

Hallux Varus: Classification and Treatment

Bernhard Devos Bevernage, MD*, Thibaut Leemrijse, MD

KEYWORDS

- Hallux varus • Classification • Osseous or ligamentous failure
- Ligamentoplasty • Dynamic and static transfers

Hallux varus deformity is generally comprised of three possible components: medial deviation of the hallux at the first metatarsophalangeal (MTP) joint, supination of the phalanx, and interphalangeal (IP) flexion or claw toe deformity.[1]

The condition can be congenital or acquired. Hallux varus is most commonly seen as an iatrogenic complication of bunion surgery, resulting from overcorrection of hallux valgus. The incidence is relatively rare, with reports ranging between 2% and 15.4% in the literature.[1–4] Iatrogenic hallux varus is often poorly tolerated.[5]

Besides iatrogenic hallux varus, several other etiologies cause acquired hallux varus: trauma, severe burn injury with contracture, systemic inflammatory disorders such as rheumatoid or psoriatic arthritis, Charcot-Marie-Tooth disease, avascular necrosis of the first metatarsal head, and paralysis or poliomyelitis.[6–9]

The goal of treatment is to obtain a functional, pain-free, shoeable foot. It is desirable to achieve a stable, aligned hallux while maintaining or maximizing joint mobility when possible.

PATHOANATOMY

The development of hallux varus is due to an imbalance between the osseous, tendon, and capsuloligamentous structures at the first MTP joint, leading to a progressive medial deviation of the great toe. This typically involves a combination of contracture or overtightening medially with excessive laxity or soft tissue attenuation laterally. In cases of iatrogenic hallux varus following bunion surgery, there may be loss of osseous support medially due to excess bone resection or an overcorrected intermetatarsal (IM) angle. Combined with excessive lateral release, such imbalance leads to unopposed pull of the medial muscles, specifically the abductor hallucis (ABH) and the medial head of the flexor hallucis brevis (FHB).

Department of Orthopaedic Surgery, Saint-Luc University Hospital, 10, Avenue Hippocrate, 1200 Brussels, Belgium
* Corresponding author.
E-mail address: bernhard.devos@uclouvain.be (B. Devos Bevernage).

Foot Ankle Clin N Am 14 (2009) 51–65
doi:10.1016/j.fcl.2008.11.007
1083-7515/08/$ – see front matter © 2009 Elsevier Inc. All rights reserved.

In order to correctly assess and treat a hallux varus deformity, one must have a thorough understanding of the contributing factors. These different factors are discussed individually below, but often exist in combination to cause the deformity. This review focuses on iatrogenic hallux varus following bunion surgery, but the same principles apply to other causes of acquired hallux varus.

Loss of Osseous Support

With excessive resection of the medial eminence or loss of a part of the tibial sesamoid groove, the medial buttress stabilizing the tibial sesamoid is lost. This results in medial drift of the tibial sesamoid and the proximal phalanx. The displacement of the tibial sesamoid out from under the first metatarsal head will further accentuate the medially deforming pull of the FHB.[1,2,7,9–12]

Excision of the Fibular Sesamoid

This compromises the stability of the plantar lateral joint structures, removing the fulcrum on which the lateral head of the FHB plantar flexes the lateral part of the proximal phalanx. This instability, in addition to other factors, may predispose to dorsiflexion of the proximal phalanx and clawing of the toe.[1,2,4,9,10,12–14]

Muscle Imbalance at the Proximal Phalangeal Base

Release or attenuation of both the adductor hallucis and the lateral head of the FHB, compounded by a release of the lateral capsule, can lead to imbalance of the MTP joint. The intact or tight medial tendons will gradually migrate more medially, increasing their deforming forces. When the center of the phalangeal base shifts medial to the midline of the first metatarsal head, the extensor hallucis longus (EHL) tendon bowstrings and pulls the toe into varus and extension. The flexor hallucis longus (FHL) will then produce a flexion at the IP joint, resulting in a claw toe.[2,7,9,10,12,15]

Overcorrection of the Intermetatarsal Angle

This typically occurs after first metatarsal osteotomy but can also occur with a purely soft tissue release, especially if the released adductor hallucis tendon is too tightly reattached to the metatarsal head. As the IM angle decreases and becomes neutral or even negative, the force vector of the medial soft tissues leads to varus position of the hallux.[1–3,7,9,10,12]

Overcorrection of Hallux Valgus Interphalangeus

Excessive medial closing wedge (Akin) phalangeal osteotomy can result in overcorrection. Due to the malposition of the phalanx, both the EHL and FHL tendons will have a medially directed force, leading to a varus position of the great toe.[1]

Excessive Medial Capsulorrhaphy

If one plicates the medial capsule too tightly, the hallux can sublux medially.[1–3,7,9,10,12]

Aggressive Postoperative Bandaging

Excessive medially oriented postoperative dressing will hold the toe malpositioned and allow for fibrosis and scarring in an adducted position.

Once the varus deformity is initiated, one can expect deterioration with time. The deformity tends to become self-perpetuating due to the medial pull of the muscles of the hallux acting at the concave side of the deformity.[2,10]

CLINICAL EVALUATION

The diagnosis of hallux varus is primarily based on clinical observation. The appearance of the toe may range from the hallux being simply "too straight" to gross medial deviation. It is crucial to determine if the deformities of the MTP and IP joints are flexible or rigid. Flexible deformities allow passive reduction, while rigid deformities result from longstanding contractures and are nonreducible. Additional components of the deformity include supination of the hallux and extension of the proximal phalanx (**Fig. 1**). Painful motion or crepitus of the MTP joint may indicate underlying arthritis and should be assessed holding the hallux in a reduced position. In long-standing deformities, the toe may not purchase the ground due to a dorsal contracture at the MTP joint, with or without flexion contracture at the IP joint. Dorsal clavus or callus at the IP joint may also be seen. The EHL tendon may be so taut that it appears in marked relief under the contracted skin.

RADIOGRAPHIC FINDINGS

Radiographic evaluation is necessary to identify the components of the deformity. Anteroposterior and lateral standing as well as complementary oblique radiographs are needed for proper evaluation. An axial sesamoid radiograph aids in assessing the sesamoid position and identify metatarsosesamoid joint arthritis (**Fig. 2**).

The hallux varus angle is formed between the longitudinal axis of the first metatarsal and the longitudinal axis of the proximal phalanx. In normal feet, this angle ranges from 5° to 15°; this will measure 0° or negative in cases of hallux varus.

Radiographs are also evaluated for potential contributing factors:

- Excessive medial eminence resection
- Medial subluxation of the tibial sesamoid out of its sesamoid groove

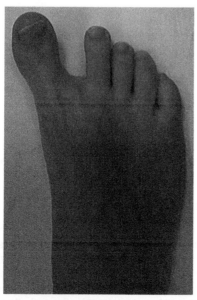

Fig. 1. An AP clinical picture of a hallux varus deformity showing the medial deviation of the hallux onto the first metatarsal and the supination of the toe, particularly visible at the toenail.

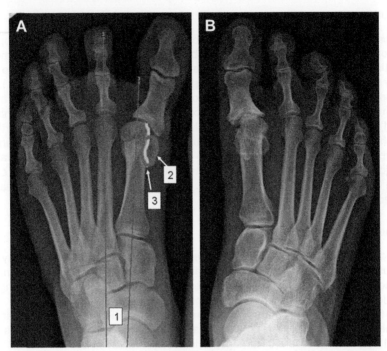

Fig. 2. (*A*) Radiographic illustration of a more or less painless, mobile first MTP joint with standing AP view: 1, intermetatarsal angle approaching 0°; 2, medial subluxation of the tibial sesamoid; 3, excessive medial eminence resection. (*B*) Radiographic example of a stiff, painful arthritic first MTP joint.

- Absence of the fibular sesamoid
- Overcorrection of the IM angle, with the angle approaching 0° or negative values
- First metatarsal longer than second metatarsal
- Phalangeal varus or malunion from prior phalangeal osteotomy
- Degenerative changes at the MTP and IP joints

The standing lateral radiograph may demonstrate dorsiflexion of the proximal phalanx at the MTP joint, with or without concomitant plantar flexion of the IP joint.

Adjunctive imaging with CT or MRI scanning is typically not required. In rare cases, these may be useful to show evidence of osteonecrosis of the first metatarsal, excessive bone resection of the metatarsal head, or arthritic involvement of the metatarso-sesamoid articulation.

NONOPERATIVE TREATMENT

Whether hallux varus is tolerated depends on how quickly it has developed, whether the joint deformities are flexible or rigid, and whether there is associated arthritis of the MTP or IP joints. Early recognition of iatrogenic hallux varus is important. If hallux varus is recognized early after bunion correction, frequent taping of the hallux into valgus position may correct the deformity. Treatment must begin as early as possible within the first few weeks and should be maintained for 3 months to allow soft tissue healing.

A fairly straight or mild flexible hallux varus can still be accommodated by wearing shoes with a wide toe box. Padding devices may cushion the toe within the shoe and prevent formation of painful calluses. When the deformity becomes severe or rigid, it poses difficulty with wearing shoes and becomes more painful. Anti-inflammatory medications may relieve pain particularly in the presence of arthritis.

CLASSIFICATION AND SURGICAL DECISION MAKING

Because of the different factors involved in the physiopathology, classification of hallux varus is a challenging endeavor. A classification scheme based solely on rigid versus flexible deformities would be overly simplistic. It is equally important to consider the presence of IP joint contracture, rotational deformity, arthritis, and bony deformity.

Certain elements must be considered in an attempt to systematically assess a hallux varus deformity for possible surgical treatment (**Table 1**). It is also crucial to consider the patient's expectations, compliance, ability to undergo complex revision surgery, and potential acceptance of joint-sacrificing options such as arthrodesis.

The first element to consider is the mobility and flexibility of the first MTP joint. In cases of severe stiffness or painful arthritis, an arthrodesis of this joint offers the most appropriate solution. If the first MTP joint remains mobile with painless motion in the reduced position, the choice of treatment will depend on associated pathologies of the IP joint and the neighboring rays.

When the hallux varus deformity has become chronically stiff and presents a fixed hammertoe deformity, demonstrates excesssive medial eminence resection, or if either articular surface has been resected in an older patient, arthrodesis of the first MTP joint along with a joint release or interposition arthroplasty of the IP joint is

Table 1
Surgical guidelines according to pain and flexibility at the MTP1 and IP joint

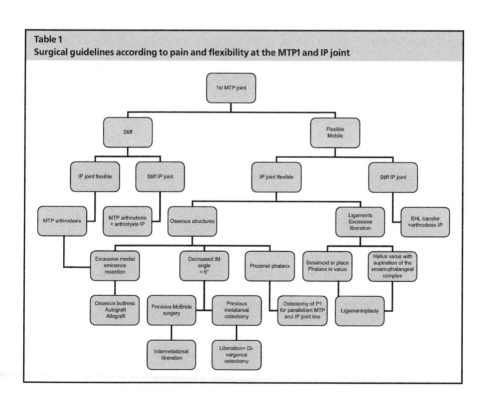

indicated. A stiff IP joint with a flexible MTP joint can be addressed by a medial release combined with EHL tendon transfer and IP arthrodesis.

When both the MTP and IP joints remain flexible, different elements contributing to the varus position must be analyzed, including the osseous structures, ligament insufficiencies, and tendon contractures.

Relevant osseous factors include excessive medial eminence resection, a decreased IM angle, and malunion of a proximal phalangeal osteotomy. Excessive bone resection at the medial aspect of the metatarsal head removes the osseous support of the tibial sesamoid as well as of the proximal phalanx. With good MTP motion in the absence of arthritis, restoration of the osseous buttress can be considered with an autograft or allograft.

Overcorrection of the IM angle following bunion surgery must be recognized. This can be due to a metatarsal osteotomy with overcorrection or due to soft tissue release of the first web space causing a lateral force vector of the phalanx against the first metatarsal closing down the first interspace. If there is overcorrection of the IM angle caused by metatarsal osteotomy, the surgeon must consider revising the osteotomy to correct alignment along with release of scar tissue and repair of the lateral ligaments. This soft tissue procedure alone may be sufficient if no metatarsal osteotomy malunion exists. The need for the revision osteotomy can be determined by a simulated weight bearing fluoroscopic image to assess the IM angle after the release of scar tissue.

Varus malunion of a proximal phalangeal (Akin) osteotomy can be reversed by a lateral closing wedge osteotomy. The purpose of such a phalangeal osteotomy is to restore parallelism between the MTP and IP joint lines, as well as to equalize the length of the hallux and the second toe.

Among the soft tissue deficits, two subtypes of excessive release of the lateral structures may exist. Both include attenuation or overly aggressive release of the lateral capsule and ligaments including the suspensory metatarsosesamoid ligament. The two subtypes can be further differentiated on standard weight bearing anteroposterior X-ray (**Fig. 3**):

- Phalangeal varus with the sesamoid bones in good position: this is most likely due to an aggressive release distal to the sesamoids.
- Hallux varus with supination taking place in the sesamoidophalangeal apparatus: this implies not only an excessive release of the lateral ligaments but also a section of the adductor tendon, as can be seen in case of fibular sesamoidectomy. This may lead to more severe instability that might necessitate an arthrodesis.

Reconstruction of these lateral components of the MTP joint can then be considered with the use of dynamic or static transfers.

OPERATIVE TREATMENTS

Numerous surgical procedures have been described for the treatment of hallux varus. Their common goal is to correct the deformity, to relieve pain, and to restore function of the forefoot. Regardless of other associated components, the first step consists of a wide capsular release on the medial aspect of the first MTP joint. As postulated by Granberry,[16] we believe the initial deforming force to be the pull of the abductor hallucis tendon. The abductor hallucis tendon insertion can be maintained or alternatively released so as to utilize the tendon for a transfer as described below.

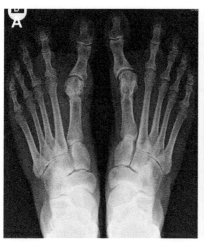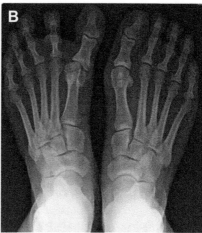

Fig. 3. (*A*) Radiograph of a standing AP view showing a hallux varus with the sesamoid bones "in place," and P1 in varus: this is most likely due to an aggressive release, distal to the sesamoids. (*B*) Radiograph of a standing AP view showing a hallux varus with some supination taking place in the sesamoidophalangeal apparatus. This image indicates not only an excessive section of the lateral collateral ligament but also a section of the adductor tendon, as can be seen in case of fibular sesamoidectomy.

Intermetatarsal Release

The first interspace must be exposed to resect the fibrosis in the intermetatarsal area. The purpose is to restore divergence between the first and second metatarsals. A separate incision in the first web space is necessary for this release. It is seldom necessary to subperiosteally free up the distal half of the first metatarsal, as proposed by Wood.[17] In practical terms, this procedure must be performed until the phalanx can be passively positioned in 10° to 15° of valgus on the first metatarsal head.

According to the preoperative clinical and radiologic assessment, the medial soft-tissue release will then be combined with either a joint conserving or joint sacrificing procedure.

In case of joint sparing surgery, additional procedures are necessary to maintain correction of the toe because medial release and first web space debridement alone do not entirely correct the deformity.[1,13,18,19] The goal is to restore physiologic valgus and to prevent recurrence of varus. One can distinguish between dynamic tendon transfers and static tendon transfers, each aiming to substitute for the incompetent lateral collateral ligament.

Dynamic Transfers

Medial release combined with adductor tendon reattachment

This may be difficult in cases of previous McBride-type surgery for hallux valgus, in which the conjoined tendon of the adductor hallucis (ADH) and the lateral head of the flexor hallucis brevis (FHB) is detached from its insertion onto the lateral sesamoid. Retraction of the muscle may preclude effective repair back to the phalangeal base (**Fig. 4**).[2,10,13]

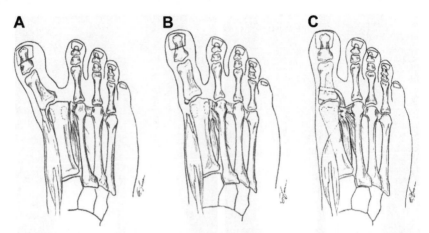

Fig. 4. Schematic diagram illustrating the medial release combined with adductor tendon reattachment. (*A*) Preoperative anatomic situation with the intermetatarsal ligament as well as the adductor hallucis tendon (oblique and transverse component) detached from the fibular sesamoid; retraction on the medial side of the varus deformity. (*B*) Medial release and adductor tendon reattachment onto the lateral sesamoid; some varus remains in the MTP1 joint which will be addressed by (*C*) an associated dynamic Hawkins transfer of the abductor hallucis tendon. (*Courtesy of* C. Husson, Brussels, Belgium.)

Medial release combined with transfer of the extensor hallucis longus tendon, with or without an interphalangeal arthrodesis

The principle is to redirect the deforming extensor hallucis longus tendon so that it exerts a correcting force: instead of dorsiflexing the MTP joint, it becomes a plantar flexor of the phalanx with a more lateral lever arm. After detaching its distal insertion, the tendon is redirected beneath the first intermetatarsal ligament to be reattached on the plantar-lateral aspect of the proximal phalanx of the great toe through a vertical tunnel. Johnson[20] reports on 15 feet surgically treated, with 14 good clinical results.

This technique relies on the intermetatarsal ligament to act as a pulley for the transferred tendon. If this ligament was sectioned during prior bunion surgery, the tendon is passed deep to a mass of scar tissue which may be unreliable to restrain the transposed tendon. According to Johnson,[20] the prior surgical scar in this region has never interfered with use of the ligament as a suitable pulley.

If the entire EHL tendon is transferred, it is necessary to fuse the IP joint to prevent a flail deformity. IP arthrodesis may be contraindicated if there is coexisting MTP stiffness and arthritis. To prevent the need for IP arthrodesis, a modification using a split EHL tendon for transfer has been proposed (**Fig. 5**).[7,21,22]

The theoretical basis for this modification was to utilize an intrinsic foot muscle rather than an extrinsic one, whose more remote muscle belly might make proper tensioning and rotational control more difficult.[1–3,6,10,14,20,23]

Medial release combined with the transfer of the first dorsal interosseous muscle

This technique was described in 1991 by Valtin,[24] who detached the distal insertion from the base of the phalanx of the second toe and transferred it through an osseous tunnel in the base of the proximal phalanx of the hallux. This creates an efficient valgus force, but the long-term effect on the second toe, deprived of its interosseous muscle, is not yet known. Furthermore, the tendon for transplantation often can be small, making reinsertion technically difficult (**Fig. 6**).[10,24]

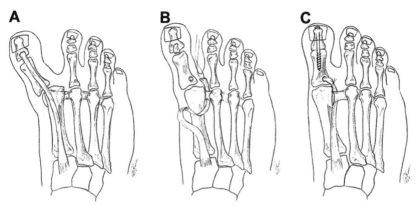

Fig. 5. Schematic diagram illustrating the medial release combined with transfer of the extensor hallucis longus (EHL) tendon, whether associated or not with an IP arthrodesis. (*A*) Preoperative anatomic situation with bowstringing of the EHL tendon at the concave, re-tracted side of the deformity. (*B*) After the necessary medial and first web space release, the varus deformity becomes passively reducible. We perform a dorso-plantar vertical tunnel at the proximal lateral basis of P1 and we harvest the EHL tendon at its insertion at P2 of the hallux. This transplant is then tagged into the first web space and passed underneath the in-termetatarsal ligament. (*C*) After recovering the transplant, it is passed from plantar to dorsal through the osseous tunnel in P1 and sutured on itself, while tensioning the transfer into a physiologic valgus position. An IP arthrodesis is performed. (*Courtesy of* C. Husson, Brussels, Belgium.)

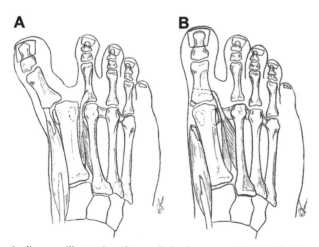

Fig. 6. Schematic diagram illustrating the medial release combined with the transfer of the first dorsal interosseous tendon. (*A*) Preoperative anatomic situation with the abductor hal-lucis tendon on the medial retracted side and the first dorsal interosseous muscle in the first web space with its tendon passing dorsally of the intermetatarsal ligament. (*B*) The essential medial release associated with the transfer of the interosseous tendon through an osseous tunnel in P1. Note the passage of the transplant dorsal from the intermetatarsal ligament. (*Courtesy of* C. Husson, Brussels, Belgium.)

Medial release combined with a transfer of the abductor hallucis tendon on the lateral base of the proximal phalanx

This technique, first described in 1971, has long been a commonly accepted procedure to correct this deformity.[4] In our experience, this tendon exhibits insufficient length in some cases, causing technical difficulties. Dissection in the first web space allows the tendon to pass plantar to the intermetatarsal ligament. The insertion on the base of the phalanx as well as the direction of the transfer will thus be plantar and may be responsible for residual phalangeal supination. This technique can be combined with the reattachment or reefing of the conjoined tendon in the web space (**Fig. 7**). [2,4,10–13,16,23,25] It is unclear if these transfers truly act in dynamic fashion. Additionally, their durability over time may diminish due to stretching out of the transfer. Consequently, a static transfer may be desirable.

Static Transfers

Medial release combined with a reversed abductor hallucis tendon transfer

After a wide medial capsular release, one third of the width of the abductor hallucis tendon is harvested from proximal to distal, keeping its distal attachment to the phalanx intact. The connecting fibers between the ABH tendon and the tibial sesamoid are sectioned. Two bone tunnels are drilled, one in the proximal phalanx and one in the metatarsal head. First, the tendon is than passed through the phalangeal tunnel from medial to lateral and recovered in the first web space. The tendon is then pulled through the metatarsal tunnel from lateral to medial and secured to the periosteum of the first metatarsal and to the remaining fibers of the ABH.

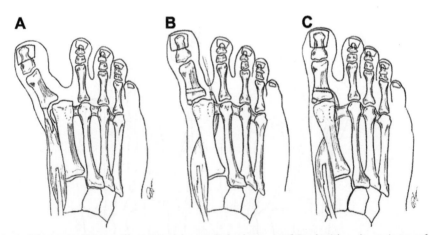

Fig. 7. Schematic diagram illustrating the medial release combined with a dynamic transfer of the abductor hallucis (ABH) tendon. (*A*) Preoperative anatomic situation showing the retraction on the medial side with the ABH tendon participating in the pathogenesis. (*B*) During the medial release, we detach the ABH tendon from its insertion onto P1 and from its adherences to the first metatarsal head and the tibial sesamoid. We create an osseous tunnel in P1 from distal medial to proximal lateral. The transplant is than passed underneath the first metatarsal and the intermetatarsal ligament. (*C*) Suture of the transplant in the corrected valgus position after passage through the tunnel. (*Courtesy of* C. Husson, Brussels, Belgium.)

The advantage of this technique is the physiologic and anatomic reconstruction of the deformity. The tendon is no longer causing the deformity and is used as an anatomic reconstruction of the lateral capsular ligament. Both the phalangeal and metatarsal tunnels are drilled closer to the center of rotation of the first MTP joint, which increases its stabilizing effect. All other functional tendons are left intact.

The authors have observed that in seven cases, the intermetatarsal angle returned to normal values, as did the tibial sesamoid position, the MTP angle and the first to second head distance (**Fig. 8**).[10]

Medial release combined with a modified split extensor hallucis longus tendon transfer

Lau and Myerson[26] note that when tension is applied distally to the lateral portion of the EHL tendon, this may statically constrain the remaining medial half of the EHL tendon. This can cause the tendon to bowstring, diminishing its excursion. They instead recommend detaching the lateral half of the EHL tendon proximally, and passing it from distal to proximal under the intermetatarsal ligament of the first web

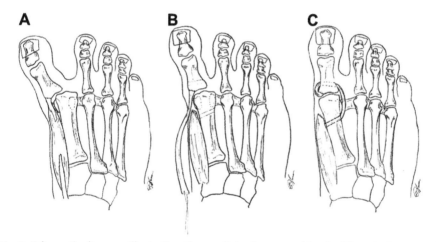

A   **B**   **C**

Fig. 8. Schematic diagram illustrating the medial release combined with a static reversed abductor hallucis (ABH) tendon transfer. (*A*) Preoperative anatomic situation with the re-tracted ABH muscle and tendon unit. (*B*) By a medial approach, a large and essential release of the first MTP joint space is realized. A third of the width of the ABH tendon is harvested from proximal to distal, keeping its insertion on the base of P1. The fibers connecting the ABH tendon and the tibial sesamoid must be released. Another incision in the first web space is then performed to realize the passage of the transplant. Two tunnels, slightly obli-que, are created: the tunnel in P1 starts some millimeters distally from the insertion of the ABH tendon and finds its way out on the lateral proximal part of P1. Both tunnels must be perfectly centered on the neutral line in order to prevent any pronation or supination of the phalanx at the moment of tightening up of the transplant. (*C*) The transplant is first passed through the tunnel in P1, recovered and tagged in the first web space and torn without twisting through the metatarsal tunnel. The transplant is next sutured with a slight tension and slight valgus of 10° to 15° by using a transosseous nonabsorbable suture, holding on to the remaining fibers of the ABH tendon. Postoperative care consists in wearing an orthopaedic shoe without weight bearing of the forefoot for 6 weeks. Mobilization of the first ray was started during the first days. A syndactyly with Elastoplast® between first and second toe must be maintained for 2 months. (*Courtesy of* C. Husson, Brussels, Belgium.)

space. As the distal attachment of the transplant is almost 2 cm away of the center of rotation of the first MTP joint, this tenodesis tends to have a supinating effect while laterally deviating the hallux (**Fig. 9**).[1,26,27]

Medial release combined with a extensor hallucis longus tenodesis

This surgical procedure resembles the previous static transfer. The EHB tendon is transferred deep to the intermetatarsal ligament and secured proximally. Again, the distal insertion of the EHB tendon is dorsal, which may lead to some supination when the transfer is tensioned (**Fig. 10**).

Ligamentoplasty

Artificial or allograft ligamentoplasties of the lateral collateral ligament have been proposed as an alternative to use of autologous tendon transfers. The below techniques attempt to induce fibrosis and stabilize the sesamoid apparatus. The disadvantages include the cost of such artificial or allograft reconstructions, ill-defined long-term results, and the potential risk of infectious transmission with allograft.[7,28]

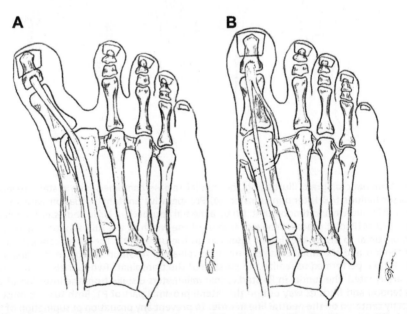

A   **B**

Fig. 9. Schematic diagram illustrating the medial release combined with a modified split extensor hallucis longus (EHL) tendon transfer. (*A*) Preoperative anatomic situation with bowstringing of the EHL tendon at the concave, retracted side of the deformity. The course of the abductor hallucis muscle is shown. (*B*) Essential medial and first web space release. The lateral half of the EHL tendon is harvested, preserving its insertion on P2. The transplant is passed underneath the intermetatarsal ligament and tagged medially through an osseous tunnel in the neck of the first metatarsal. Suture is performed holding to hallux in the corrected position. (*Courtesy of* C. Husson, Brussels, Belgium.)

A   **B**   **C**

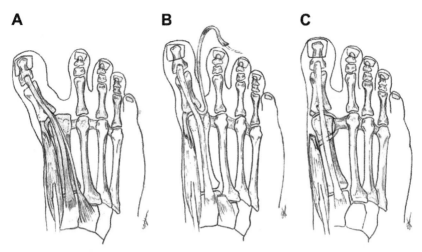

Fig. 10. Schematic diagram illustrating the medial release combined with an extensor hallucis brevis (EHB) tenodesis. (*A*) Preoperative anatomic situation with bowstringing of the extensor hallucis longus tendon at the concave, retracted side of the deformity. The course of the EHB tendon and the abductor hallucis muscle are depicted. (*B*) After the essential medial release, the tendon of the EHB is harvested by a stab incision, while it remains inserted onto the dorsolateral basis of P1. The transplant is passed underneath the intermetatarsal ligament and through an oblique osseous tunnel starting just proximal and lateral of the head of the first metatarsal to end more proximally of the medial vascular bundle entering the first metatarsal head. (*C*) The transplant is then sutured while maintaining the hallux in a physiologic, congruent valgus position. (*Courtesy of* C. Husson, Brussels, Belgium.)

The techniques are:

1. Medial release combined with the Saragaglia's technique[19] of reconstruction of the lateral ligament using Ligapro suture.
2. Medial release combined with the reinforcement of the lateral capsular ligament by the use of fascia lata, or associated with capsular repair using a soft-tissue anchor.[15,18]

Osseous Buttress

In cases of a flexible hallux varus deformity that is due to an overresection of the medial metatarsal head, a bone graft is used to reconstitute the medial metatarsal head. The graft is secured with screws and may help restore normal kinematics of the first MTP joint. It restores support for the tibial sesamoid to prevent medial subluxation and also buttresses the base of the proximal phalanx. This stabilization of the MTP joint is believed to restore the interaction of the intrinsic and extrinsic muscles in a more neutral axis. Originally described by Roy-Camille and colleagues,[29] Rochwerger and colleagues[11] noticed persisting satisfying results in 10 patients, even after 22 year (mean 8.6 years).

All these surgical procedures may be combined, if needed (**Fig. 11**).

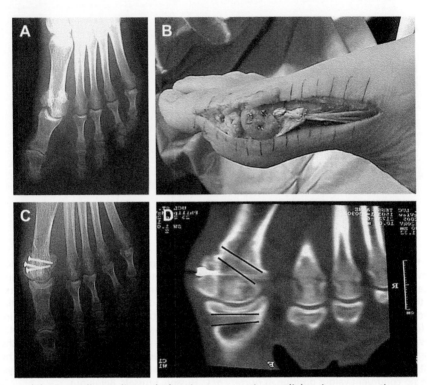

Fig. 11. (*A*) AP standing radiograph showing an excessive medial eminence resection, associated with an aggressive lateral release distal to the sesamoids, after failed hallux valgus surgery. The first MTP joint is mobile, reducible, and painless. (*B*) Intraoperative view with nice correction into a physiologic valgus position, illustrating the combination of an osseous allograft buttress and a static reversed abductor hallucis tendon transfer. (*C*) Postoperative AP standing radiograph at 2-year follow-up. (*D*) CT scan illustrating the persistence of the osseous trajectory of the tendinous transplant as well as the osteo-integration of the allograft buttress with the metatarsal head.

SUMMARY

Most of the literature on the treatment of hallux varus consists of Level IV retrospective case series. Comparison between different techniques is therefore quite difficult, particularly in view of the various contributing factors involved. Appropriate treatment requires careful clinical and radiographic assessment to identify the involved factors. These are then addressed to correct all elements of the deformity.

REFERENCES

1. Groulier P, Curvale G. [Postoperative iatrogenic hallux varus. Surgical treatment] [French]. Rev Chir Orthop Reparatrice Appar Mot 1992;78:449–55.
2. Edelman RD. Iatrogenically induced hallux varus. Clin Podiatr Med Surg 1991;8: 367–82.
3. Goldman FD, Siegel J. Extensor hallucis longus tendon transfer for correction of hallux varus. J Foot Ankle Surg 1993;32:126–31.
4. Hawkins FB. Acquired hallux valgus: cause, prevention and correction. Clin Orthop Relat Res 1971;76:169–76.

5. Trnka H-J, Zettl R. Acquired hallux varus and clinical tolerability. Foot Ankle Int 1997;18:593–7.
6. Davies M, Parker B. Idiopathic hallux varus. Foot Ankle Int 1995;16:210–1.
7. Donley BG. Acquired hallux varus. Foot Ankle Int 1997;18:586–92.
8. Saraiya H. Case report: post-burn hallux varus: a case report and management of a rare deformity. Burns 2000;26:593–8.
9. Vanore J, Christensen J. Diagnosis and treatment of first metatarsophalangeal joint disorders. Section 3: hallux varus. J Foot Ankle Surg 2003;42:137–42.
10. Leemrijse Th, Hoang B, Maldague P, et al. A new surgical procedure for iatrogenic hallux varus: Reverse transfer of the abductor hallucis tendon. A report of 7 cases. Acta Orthop Belg 2008;74:227–34.
11. Rochwerger A, Curvale G, Groulier P. Application of bone graft to the medial side of the first metatarsal head in the treatment of hallux varus. J Bone Joint Surg Am 1999;81:1730–5.
12. Zahari D, Girolamo M. Hallux varus: a step-wise approach for correction. J Foot Surg 1991;30:264–6.
13. Jahss MH. Spontaneous hallux varus: relation to poliomyelitis and congenital absence of the fibular sesamoid. Foot Ankle 1983;3:224–6.
14. Turner RS. Dynamic post-surgical hallux varus after lateral sesamoidectomy: treatment and prevention. Orthopedics 1986;9:963–9.
15. Labovitz JM, Kaczander BI. Traumatic hallux varus repair utilizing a soft-tissue anchor: a case report. J Foot Ankle Surg 2000;39:120–3.
16. Granberry WM, Hickey CH. Idiopathic adult hallux valgus. Foot Ankle Int 1994;15:197–205.
17. Wood WA. Acquired hallux varus; a new corrective procedure. J Foot Surg 1981;20:194–7.
18. Stanifer E, Hodor D. Congenital hallux varus: case presentation and review of the literature. J Foot Surg 1991;30:509–12.
19. Tourné Y, Saragaglia D. Iatrogenic hallux varus surgical procedure: a study of 14 cases. Foot Ankle Int 1995;16:457–63.
20. Johnson KA, Spiegl PV. Extensor hallucis longus transfer for hallux varus deformity. J Bone Joint Surg 1984;66:681–6.
21. Hunter WN, Wasiak GA. Traumatic hallux varus correction via split extensor tenodesis. J Foot Surg 1984;23:321–5.
22. Katz JB. Correction of hallux varus via split tendon transfer. J Am Podiatry Assoc 1990;80:498–501.
23. Maynou C, Beltrand E. [Tendon transfers in postoperative hallux varus] [French]. Rev Chir Orthop Reparatrice Appar Mot 2000;86:181–7.
24. Valtin B. [First dorsal interosseous muscle transfer in iatrogenic hallux varus surgery] [French]. Med Chir Pied 1991;7:9–16.
25. Clark WD. Abductor hallucis tendon transfer for hallux varus. J Foot Surg 1984;23:146–8.
26. Lau J, Myerson M. Technique tip: modified split extensor hallucis longus tendon transfer for correction of hallux varus. Foot Ankle Int 2002;23:1138–40.
27. Mann R. Comment on: modified split extensor hallucis longus tendon transfer for correction of hallux varus. Foot Ankle Int 2004;25:43.
28. Myerson MS, Komenda GA. Results of hallux varus correction using an extensor hallucis brevis tenodesis. Foot Ankle Int 1996;17:21–7.
29. Roy-Camille R, Lelievre JF. [Treatment of hypercorrection after surgical procedure on hallux valgus. Medial osteoplastic ridge] [French]. Nouv Presse Med 1978;28:3357–8.

Nerve Disorders of the Hallux

Stuart D. Miller, MD

KEYWORDS

• Causalgia • Hallux • Innervations • Neuritis • Sclerosing

The hallux plays an important role in standing and walking and thus has elaborate innervation. The superficial location of the nerves innervating the hallux predisposes to injury or damage that can have significant impact on ambulatory ability. The disability caused by nerve pain should not be underestimated, as even a small peripheral nerve can cause enough disruption within the nervous system to generate a complex regional pain syndrome or causalgia, with potentially catastrophic results.[1] This article discusses nerve pathology of the hallux, including the superficial peroneal nerve (SPN), the deep peroneal nerve (DPN), and hallucal branches of the medial plantar nerve.

ANATOMY

The anatomy of the cutaneous innervation of the hallux can be confusing. The patterns of innervation can be variable and may not adhere to textbook descriptions. The plantar surface is innervated by branches of the medial plantar nerve, while the dorsum receives the terminal aspects of the superficial and deep peroneal nerves (**Fig. 1**). The most detailed text on anatomy of the foot describes several patterns of first web space innervation.[2] Historically, confusion arose because one prominent surgical anatomy atlas drew the saphenous nerve supplying the medial aspect of the toe, a situation not seen clinically.[3] Instead, the medial aspect of the dorsal hallux is innervated by the terminal branch of the superficial peroneal nerve, sometimes with a contribution from the deep peroneal nerve. Despite anatomic variations, most innervation patterns can be elucidated with careful examination and local anesthetic blocks.

NONOPERATIVE APPROACH TO NEURITIS

Initial evaluation and treatment of nerve disorders of the foot usually follow a similar pattern. The patient is questioned about medical comorbidities, trauma history, prior foot or ankle surgeries, and the location, severity, and character of the symptoms. Examination begins with observing the skin for any scars, prior burns, or contractures that

Department of Orthopaedic Surgery, Union Memorial Hospital, 3333 North Calvert Street, Suite 400, Baltimore, MD 21218, USA
E-mail address: stubonedoc@aol.com

Foot Ankle Clin N Am 14 (2009) 67–75
doi:10.1016/j.fcl.2008.11.010
1083-7515/08/$ – see front matter © 2009 Elsevier Inc. All rights reserved.

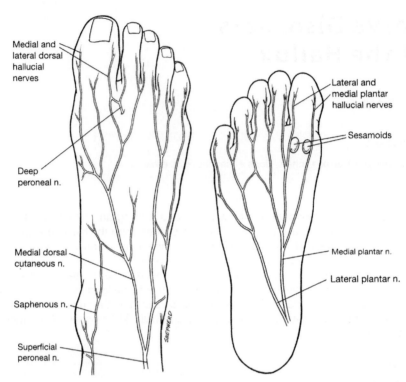

Fig. 1. Dorsal and plantar sensory nerve anatomy to the great toe. (*Reproduced from* Bowman MW. Athletic injuries of the great toe MTP joint. In: Adelar RS, editor. Complete foot and ankle trauma. Philadelphia: Lippincott-Raven; 1999. p. 238; with permission.)

could suggest entrapment of the cutaneous nerves. Overall alignment of the foot and the hallux is assessed. The location of tenderness is determined along with identification of any bony osteophytes on the foot or about the hallux. It is important to assess the degree of sensory impairment to light touch and with more detailed monofilament testing. Hypesthesias and dysesthesias are identified and percussion test (Tinel's sign) is carefully performed for the different nerve branches around the ankle, midfoot, and hallux. Careful consideration of the underlying innervation anatomy can assist the examiner in determining the involved nerve(s). The patient's gait is observed for any gross malalignment or dynamic deformities. The patient's shoewear should be inspected for any sites of potential mechanical compression. Standing radiographs can help to rule out osteophytes or bone deformities which might cause nerve irritation or impingement.

Nonoperative treatment focuses on relieving pain, maintaining function, and preventing deconditioning. Physical therapy modalities can help break down scar tissue and aid with desensitization of neuritis symptoms. Therapeutic exercise can prevent stiffness, weakness, and dysfunction of the limb. Local anesthetic injection is helpful for both diagnostic and therapeutic purposes. An injection of lidocaine and bupivicaine (with a drop or two of sodium bicarbonate added to diminish stinging) is placed adjacent to the affected nerve at a level proximal to the area of symptoms. Temporary relief of symptoms and normalization of Tinel's sign helps to confirm the diagnosis. The surgeon should reexamine the patient 5 to 10 minutes after the injection to discern the efficacy of the local block.

The primary goal of pharmacologic treatment is to lower the amplitude of nerve irritation and reduce symptoms. Many patients respond to nerve modulating medications such as gabapentin and pregabalin. Amytriptyline in low doses nightly can be helpful, especially when sleep cycles are disrupted. Clonazopine also seems to help some patients. Unfortunately the central nervous system side effects of these medications often limit their applicability. Anti-inflammatory medications may provide some analgesia, while narcotics are used sparingly. Pain management specialists are extremely helpful in managing these multimodality medication regimens.

Local pharmacologic treatment can often provide some relief. Lidoderm pads are self-adherent foam pads impregnated with lidocaine hydrochloride which leech transdermally over several hours, anesthetizing the affected nerve locally. Another topical treatment involves a gel compound containing pain and nerve medications which can be compounded in a local pharmacy. A prescription for gabapentin, lidocaine, amytriptyline, and other medications can allow the pharmacist to create a gel mixture which can be applied topically; the efficacy of these agents remains to be clearly defined in this complicated population.

Sclerosing injections are a reasonable alternative to surgical treatment. The nerve is injected with a solution of 4% ethanol in bupivicaine hydrochloride to cause chemical damage to the nerve; this technique has been used for interdigital neuromas, with anecdotal success rates of 70%.[4] Initial nerve block with local anesthetic must be successful for the surgeon to consider the sclerosing treatment regimen. The regimen consists of four injections spaced 7 to 10 days apart, followed by three more injections if the initial series is successful but relief of symptoms is limited in duration. There seem to be few contraindications for sclerosing injections other than localized hypersensitivity or preexisting complex regional pain syndrome, which could possibly be exacerbated by the nerve irritation. No clear pattern of tissue damage as a result of the sclerosing treatments has been demonstrated at subsequent surgical resection.

SURGICAL TREATMENT OF NERVE DISORDERS

Surgical treatment for nerve problems follows simple guidelines whenever possible. A positive nerve block helps to confirm the diagnosis and should be a precursor to most surgical interventions. If an offending bone prominence or malalignment exists, then bony correction may help the neuritis. In cases of nerve entrapment, stenosis, or traction injury, neurolysis and decompression can relieve symptoms. Neurolysis offers little improvement, however, if the surgeon encounters minimal scar tissue or entrapment of the nerve (the efficacy of neurolysis in such circumstances has not been noted in the literature). Many surgeons recommend further intervention at the time of surgery if neurolysis is felt to offer little improvement or if the nerve is severely damaged, such as a prior crush injury or surgical neuroma. The nerves at the level of the hallux are all purely sensory and thus can be resected with little functional loss.

If there is a frank neuroma from prior surgery or if the nerve is severely scarred from prior crush injury, then resection with burial of the nerve stump into bone works well. Chiodo and Miller[5] report pain improvement of 5.4 points (from 8.6 to 3.2) on a 10-point visual analog scale for SPN transection and burial into bone. Sunderland[6] noted "Why some [neuromas] should be painful and others insensitive, even in the same individual, remains a mystery." The level of transection and whether to bury the stump into bone or muscle are ill-defined. A general principle would be to salvage as much nerve as possible. Controversy still lingers regarding the appropriate method of nerve transaction and whether to bury the nerve ending into bone or a muscle bed.[5,7]

DORSOMEDIAL CUTANEOUS NERVE

The dorsomedial cutaneous nerve (DMCN) is the terminal extension of the superficial peroneal nerve which innervates the dorsal and medial aspect of the hallux. (**Fig. 2**) The nerve has a variable course and intermingles with the deep peroneal nerve.[2,8,9] The superficial peroneal nerve is purely sensory and can be compressed at the distal third of the leg as it egresses from the deep muscular fascia; such compression can result in distal sensory findings similar to DMCN pathology.

Neuritis of the DMCN can occur iatrogenically following bunion surgery.[10] Almost any procedure around the hallux can damage this nerve, which may demonstrate unusual branching.[9,11] The nerve may be within the surgical field and can be damaged by retraction. An early study noted that 15 of 55 incisional neuromas in a series of foot and ankle neuromas affected the DMCN.[12] The author later found that half of the eight patients with unsatisfactory results following distal first metatarsal osteotomy had neuritic symptoms over the dorsum of the toe or at the incision site.[13,14]

Nerve compression can occur between the bony prominence of the first metatarsal head and a shoe. A careful preoperative examination should be recorded since some patients have nerve damage before any surgical intervention due to impingement on bony prominence.[15]

Decreased sensation to the great toe can also occur following ankle fracture due to more proximal injury of the superficial peroneal nerve. One study of 120 patients with ankle fractures found 15% had symptomatic injury to the SPN.[16] This included 9% of patients treated with casting and 21% treated surgically. An obvious mechanism of injury during surgery is traction injury or iatrogenic neuroma during exposure of the fibula. A more subtle injury to the nerve may result from traction to the SPN during sprain or fracture. Cadaver research documents the stretch and strain on the SPN with ankle inversion before and after transaction of the anterior talofibular ligament, noting a significant increase in nerve excursion and strain in the presence of incompetent ligaments.[17] The SPN can be compressed as the nerve exits from under the peroneal fascia in the leg; the symptoms can radiate to the dorsal foot including the hallux.[18] Yet another study documented damage to the SPN with procedures around the foot and ankle, noting varied patterns to the SPN and the obvious risk with ankle arthroscopy and arthrotomy.[19]

Treatment should proceed cautiously. In many cases, the sensory changes are temporary and nonsurgical care is recommended for 3 to 6 months. If nonsurgical treatment does not alleviate symptoms then surgery may be indicated.

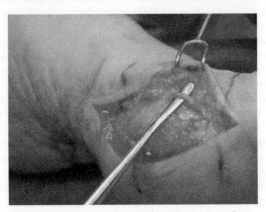

Fig. 2. The dorsomedial cutaneous nerve lies on the joint retinaculum capsule.

For the DMCN, resection and burial of the stump involves a dorsomedial incision along the course of the nerve. The nerve is resected distally in the incision and the distal ending is cauterized to prevent neurotropic hormone release. The proximal end is transected obliquely, which limits neuroma formation,[20] and then buried into the bone of the proximal metatarsal or the medial cuneiform, whichever seems most appropriate. The periosteum should be cut and then the hole drilled with a 2.5-mm drill bit. Care should be taken to protect the soft tissues, especially the nerve itself, from the drill. The nerve can then be placed into the unicortical hole and, if desired, the periosteum secured around it with one stitch. Subcutaneous suture and skin closure are performed. Postoperative wound care would allow early weight bearing with attention to limiting swelling of the foot. Desensitization exercises seem to help postoperatively. The patient should be warned that some dysesthesias can be expected in the region of the nerve distribution. A study of 10 patients documented an improvement in the 10-point visual analog scale from 2.1 to 8.6 points at an average follow-up of 22 months and that all 10 patients would undergo the surgery again.[21]

DEEP PERONEAL NERVE

The deep peroneal nerve extends along the dorsal tibia and emerges from under the superior extensor retinaculum. The patterns of innervations are variable. The nerve is primarily sensory but sends a motor branch to the extensor hallucis brevis muscle. A posterior sensory branch has also been described to the sinus tarsi region.[22] The main nerve branch runs dorsally on the midfoot and terminates in the first web space. The deep peroneal nerve is at obvious risk for mechanical trauma or iatrogenic injury with surgery of the midfoot. Compression of the deep peroneal nerve can occur from underlying synovitis or osteophytes in midfoot arthritis, or due to pressure from a ganglion cyst or varicosities. The nerve has little soft tissue coverage which means that once irritated or damaged, it often remains a source of pain. More proximally at the ankle retinaculum, an impingement syndrome has been described which can cause distal pain as well.[23] Beyond the retinaculum, the nerve can be entrapped along with the extensor hallucis muscle.[24,25] More distally, the nerve runs deep into the first web space and can be at risk with bunion surgery or with fusion procedures.

A neuroma of the DPN should also be treated nonoperatively for at least several months. The nerve may slowly recover, with or without full return of sensation. A hypoesthetic area in the first web space can be easily tolerated. With persistent symptoms, diagnostic nerve injection can be useful. Diagnostic injection on the dorsal midfoot may block the DPN or branches of the SPN, which may confuse the source of symptoms. Injection at the supramalleolar region is preferred; this is performed deep to the retinaculum between the EHL and EDL tendons. Relief of symptoms suggests that the DPN rather than the SPN is the source.

For a simple impingement syndrome, neurolysis can work very well, especially for problems with the anterior ankle retinaculum. Surgical resection of DPN neuromata has not been well documented. This author finds prolonged irritation with resection and burial along the dorsum of the foot and chooses to resect and bury the nerve at the level of the distal tibia. Unpublished data from over 25 cases of DPN resection found better clinical response than for SPN nerve resection. The reason for the good results probably stems from the proximity of the DPN to the anterior tibial bone in the distal leg.

An anterior incision can be made over the distal leg. The SPN is protected in the subcutaneous tissues and the extensor retinaculum incised longitudinally. The interval between the extensor hallucis longus and the extensor digitorum longus muscles will lead to the neurovascular bundle consisting of the DPN, the anterior tibial artery, and two large veins. The nerve can be gently separated and then the distal end obliquely transected just above the ankle. The more proximal end can be buried into the adjacent tibia. The periosteum over the tibia is incised and a 2.5-mm drill bit used to create a unicortical hole, rounding off the proximal edge to allow easy insertion of the nerve stump. The muscle fascia should be closed when possible and the patient is often immobilized in a splint for 10–14 days to allow soft tissue healing. Many patients seem to have more pain from the muscle dissection rather than the nerve transection. When concomitant SPN nerve pain is being treated, the two nerves can be resected through one long S-shaped incision.

THE MEDIAL PLANTAR NERVE

The medial plantar nerve, a branch of the posterior tibial nerve, courses deep to the abductor hallucis muscle in the foot and branches in a variable pattern to the hallux and the medial forefoot.[26,27] This nerve lies within a complicated web of tissues on the medial aspect of the foot. Surgery for transfer of the flexor hallucis longus has been noted to cause damage to the medial plantar nerve.[14,28–30] This nerve has also been injured with metatarsal shortening.[14] Iatrogenic compression of the nerve can also occur, including dynamic compression in runners or athletes during exercise. Distally, the medial plantar nerve has two branches that innervate the plantar skin under the hallux. The medial branch courses adjacent to the tibial sesamoid and is prone to injury with surgery in this region. Most surgeons recommend visualization of the nerve during surgical exposures for plantar plate repair or sesamoidectomy. The next intermediate branch of the medial plantar nerve courses directly under the lateral sesamoid; the surgeon must carefully retract this nerve during fibular sesamoid excision to prevent injury. (**Fig. 3**) Damage to these terminal branches of the medial

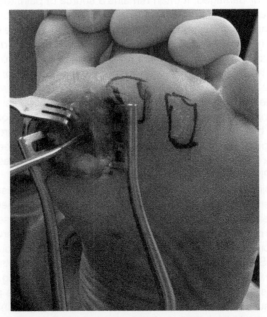

Fig. 3. The plantar nerve to the lateral aspect of the hallux, overlying the fibular sesamoid. The surgical instrument is pointing out the nerve.

plantar nerve presents a challenging treatment scenario. Nonoperative measures are attempted, especially after fibular sesamoidectomy where a slow recovery can occur over months. Medications and injections are attempted as described above. Physical therapy can facilitate movement of the toe, prevent contracture, and desensitize the tissues. Orthotic management is also warranted, consisting of an orthotic insole with a metatarsal pad and relief under the symptomatic area.

When nonoperative measures fail, a decision regarding surgical intervention hinges on the cause of the injury. The role of neurolysis has not been well defined in the literature; this author finds it of limited merit since the nerve seems to scar into very thick tissue at the distal levels. Some have reported successful nerve repair by grafting, but this treatment involves a long recovery period.[31] Surgical neuromas do well with resection and burial into the deep intrinsic musculature of the foot.[29] Resection of the medial plantar nerve involves a long incision on the plantar aspect of the foot proximal to the sesamoids. The plantar fascia is incised longitudinally and the nerve dissected free from the deep intrinsic muscles of the foot. Whereas the innervation patterns can be variable, especially with the medial branch to the first ray and the intermediate branch to the first interspace, the nerve is usually quite easily identified (**Fig. 4**A). The distal branches leading to the zone of injury are transected while preserving as much of the other (usually lateral) branches as possible. The end of the cut nerve can be buried deep into the arch of the foot, usually into the substance of the quadratus musculature (**Fig. 4**B). Although patients worry that the foot will become insensate on the plantar aspect, the adjacent plantar nerves have provided more than enough protective sensation to protect against ulceration.[29]

Nerve disorders about the hallux can generate remarkable pain and dysfunction. Whether caused by soft tissue entrapment, trauma, iatrogenic injury, or from an idiopathic basis, nerve disorders are approached by careful history and examination followed by nonoperative treatment. In cases that do not respond, meticulous surgical management can be helpful in many cases.

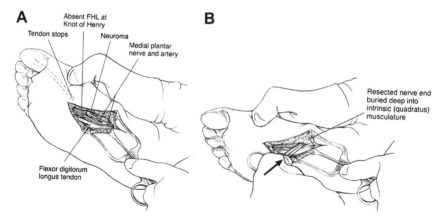

Fig. 4. (*A*) The plantar medial approach to the medial plantar nerve and branches. (*B*) Resection and burial of the transected nerve ending into the deep intrinsic musculature of the foot. (*Reproduced from* Herbst SA, Miller SD. Transection of the medial plantar nerve and hallux cock-up deformity after flexor hallucis longus transfer for Achilles tendonitis: case report. Foot Ankle Int 2006;27:640; with permission. Copyright © 2009 by the American Orthopedic Foot and Ankle Society, Inc.)

REFERENCES

1. Jupiter JB, Seiler JG, Zienowicz R. Sympathetic maintained pain (causalgia) associated with a demonstrable peripheral-nerve lesion. J Bone Joint Surg Am 1994;76(9):1376–84.
2. Sarrafian SK. Functional anatomy of the foot and ankle. In: Sarrafian SK, editor. Anatomy of the foot and ankle: descriptive, topographic, functional anatomy. 2nd edition. Philadelphia: JBLippincott; 1993. p. 474–602.
3. Hoppenfeld S, de Boer P. Surgical exposures in orthopaedics: the anatomic approach. Philadelphia: Lippincott; 1984. p. 525.
4. Dockery GL. The treatment of intermetatarsal neuromas with 4% alcohol sclerosing injections. J Foot Ankle Surg 1999;38(6):403–8.
5. Chiodo C, Miller SD. Surgical treatment of superficial peroneal neuromas. Foot Ankle Int 2004;25(10):689–94.
6. Sunderland S. Nerve injuries and their repair: a critical appraisal. Edinburgh: Churchill Livingstone; 1991.
7. Dellon AL, Aszmann OC. Treatment of superficial and deep peroneal neuromas by resection and translocation of the nerves into the anterolateral compartment. Foot Ankle Int 1998;19:300–3.
8. Miller RA, Hartman G. Origin and course of the dorsomedial cutaneous nerve to the great toe. Foot Ankle Int 1996;17(10):620–3.
9. Solan MC, Lemon M, Bendall SP. The surgical anatomy of the dorsomedial cutaneous nerve of the hallux. J Bone Joint Surg Br 2001;83(2):250–2.
10. Campbell DA. Sensory nerve damage during surgery on the hallux. J R Coll Surg Edinb 1992;37(6):422–4.
11. Canovas F, Bonnel F, Kouloumdjian P. The superficial peroneal nerve at the foot. Organisation, surgical applications. Surg Radiol Anat 1996;18(3):241–4.
12. Kenzora JE. Symptomatic incisional neuromas on the dorsum of the foot. Foot Ankle 1984;5(1):2–15.
13. Kenzora JE. Sensory nerve neuromas leading to failed foot surgery. Foot Ankle 1986;7(2):110–7.
14. Meier PJ, Kenzora JE. The risks and benefits of distal first metatarsal osteotomies. Foot Ankle 1985;6(1):7–17.
15. Herron ML, Kar S, Beard D, et al. Sensory dysfunction in the great toe in hallux valgus. J Bone Joint Surg Br 2004;86(1):54–7.
16. Redfern DJ, Suave PS, Sakellariou A. Investigation of incidence of superficial peroneal nerve injury following ankle fracture. Foot Ankle Int 2003;24(10):771–4.
17. O'Neill PJ, Parks BG, Walsh R, et al. Excursion and strain of the superficial peroneal nerve during inversion ankle sprain. J Bone Joint Surg Am 2007;89(5):979–86.
18. Styf J. Entrapment of the superficial peroneal nerve. diagnosis and results of decompression. J Bone Joint Surg Br 1989;71(1):131–5.
19. Blair JM, Botte MJ. Surgical anatomy of the superficial peroneal nerve in the ankle and foot. Clin Orthop 1994;305:229–38.
20. Marcol W, Kotulska K, Larysz-Brysz M, et al. Prevention of painful neuromas by oblique transection of peripheral nerves. J Neurosurg 2006;104(2):258–9.
21. Mohler JR, Hanel DP. Closed fractures complicated by peripheral nerve injury. J Am Acad Orthop Surg 2006;14(1):32–7.
22. Rab M, Ebmer J, Dellon AL. Innervation of the sinus tarsi and implications for treating anterolateral ankle pain. Ann Plast Surg 2001;47(5):500–4.

23. Andresen BL, Wertsch JJ, Stewart WA. Anterior tarsal tunnel syndrome. Arch Phys Med Rehabil 1992;73(11):1112–7.

24. Kanbe K, Kubota H, Shirakura K, et al. Entrapment neuropathy of the deep peroneal nerve associated with the extensor hallucis brevis. J Foot Ankle Surg 1995; 34(6):50–2.

25. Reed SC, Wright CS. Compression of the deep branch of the peroneal nerve by the extensor hallucis brevis muscle: a variation of the anterior tarsal tunnel syndrome. Can J Surg 1995;38(6):545–6.

26. Lumsden DB, Schon LC, Easley ME, et al. Topography of the distal tibial nerve and its branches. Foot Ankle Int 2003;24(9):696–700.

27. Still PG, Fowler MB. Joplin's neuroma or compression neuropathy of the plantar proper digital nerve to the hallux: clinicopathologic study of three cases. J Foot Ankle Surg 1998;37(6):524–30.

28. Frenette JP, Jackson DW. Lacerations of the flexor hallucis longus in the young athlete. J Bone Joint Surg Am 1977;59(5):673–6.

29. Herbst SA, Miller SD. Transection of the medial plantar nerve and hallux cock-up deformity after flexor hallucis longus transfer for Achilles tendonitis: case report. Foot Ankle Int 2006;27(8):639–41.

30. Mulier T, Rummens E, Dereymaker G. Risk of neurovascular injuries in flexor hallucis longus tendon transfers: an anatomic cadaver study. Foot Ankle Int 2005;28(8):910–5.

31. Kim J, Dellon AL. Reconstruction of a painful post-traumatic medial plantar neuroma with a bioabsorbable nerve conduit: a case report. J Foot Ankle Surg 2001;40(5):318–23.

First Metatarsal Malunion

Adam Becker, MD

KEYWORDS

• Cheilectomy • Hallux • Malunion • Metatarsal • Osteotomy

Malunion of a first metatarsal osteotomy or fracture can result in deformity and unloading of the first ray. The two most common deformities consist of dorsal angulation of the distal fragment and shortening of the metatarsal, although other deformities can occur. Dorsiflexion and shortening occur as a result of the net dorsiflexion force on the distal metatarsal during the foot flat and toe off portions of stance phase. This unloading of the first metatarsal can result in transfer lesions to the lesser toes. Dorsal malunion is most commonly reported after the proximal crescentic osteotomy, with a reported incidence as high as 80%.[1] Malunions can be caused by improper orientation of the osteotomy, poor intraoperative fixation, or loss of fixation postoperatively due to premature weight bearing or catastrophic failure. There is little in the literature on the rate and incidence of malunion following first metatarsal fractures treated either operatively or nonoperatively. However, treatment options would be similar as for malunion following an osteotomy. The treatment of malunions depends on how symptomatic the patient is, including pain, difficulty with ambulation, and whether they complain of transfer metatarsalgia.

DISTAL OSTEOTOMY MALUNION

Distal first metatarsal osteotomies are commonly used to correct mild-to-moderate hallux valgus deformities. Various osteotomies have been described, each with its own geometric configuration which has implications for ease of surgical technique, healing potential, and biomechanical stability. Distal osteotomies have been shown to be biomechanically more stable then proximal first metatarsal osteotomies. Shereff et al.[2–5] compared the stability of five distal first metatarsal osteotomies and one proximal osteotomy. The distal osteotomies studied include the chevron osteotomy, distal transverse osteotomy, Mitchell step-cut osteotomy, distal biplanar osteotomy, and basilar osteotomy. They conclude that the chevron osteotomy is the most stable of the distal osteotomies, with no significant difference in the stability of the remaining distal osteotomies. However, all five distal osteotomies are significantly more stable than the basilar osteotomy. Of the complications mentioned earlier, the most prevalent

Englewood Orthopedic Associates, Englewood NJ 07631, USA
E-mail address: beckerad@gmail.com

Foot Ankle Clin N Am 14 (2009) 77–90
doi:10.1016/j.fcl.2008.11.006
1083-7515/08/$ – see front matter © 2009 Elsevier Inc. All rights reserved.

with distal osteotomies are shortening, dorsal malunion, hallux varus, and avascular necrosis (AVN).

A commonly used distal osteotomy for correction of a mild-to-moderate bunion deformity is the chevron osteotomy.[6] The geometry of the osteotomy conveys some stability against sagittal plane angulation and varus/valgus instability. Dorsal malunion and shortening, however, do occur rarely following a chevron osteotomy. Once the use of fixation became popular, these complications with chevron osteotomies have decreased. Shortening is most likely secondary to the width of the saw blade used, impaction of the distal fragment, and lack of cortical support. Trnka and colleagues[7] published their clinical and radiographic results of 57 consecutive chevron osteotomies at 2 to 5 years follow-up. They report two feet (3.5%) with valgus malunions and one foot (1.7%) with a dorsal malunion.

The Mitchell osteotomy is a step-cut distal first metatarsal osteotomy also used for correction of mild-to-moderate deformities[8–10] As Shereff and colleagues[2] demonstrated, the Mitchell osteotomy lacks the stability of the chevron osteotomy. Teli and colleagues[11–15] published their experience of sixty feet treated with Mitchell osteotomies for the treatment of hallux valgus with k-wire fixation and early weightbearing. Three feet (4%) had early loss of correction, and six feet (10%) had unrelieved or new onset of metatarsalgia related to excessive shortening or malalignment of the first metatarsal. Fokter and colleagues[16] report the results after 251 Mitchell osteotomies with a mean 21-year follow up. The average shortening of the first metatarsal was 5.4 mm, with metatarsalgia and deformity recurrence as the main causes of poor results.

Transcervical distal metatarsal osteotomies have been described using both open and percutaneous techniques. Jahss[17,18] and colleagues reported good results with a biplanar neck osteotomy made perpendicular to the first metatarsal shaft allowing lateral and plantar translation of the head fragment. The percutaneous technique was first described by Bosch[19] and later popularized by Giannini for mild-to-moderate hallux valgus deformities. Portaluri[20] published his results on 143 patients treated with the Bosch technique with 89% patient satisfaction. More recently, Kadakia and Myerson and colleagues[21] reported on their early radiographic outcomes and complications of a percutaneous distal first metatarsal transverse osteotomy in 13 consecutive patients. 69% of the patients demonstrated dorsally angulated alignment of the first metatarsal of 10° on their first post-operative examination; this subsequently increased to 15.9° by final follow up, with one patient developing a frank nonunion.

DORSAL MALUNIONS AND SHORTENING

Dorsal malunions often present with complaints of pain about the first metatarsal phalangeal (MTP) joint in addition to overloading of the lesser toes secondary to offloading of the first ray. Osteotomies demonstrating shortening without dorsal angulation may present with similar symptoms. Dorsal malunions may also lead to restricted dorsiflexion of the MTP joint secondary to dorsal impingement. On examination, the posture and length of the hallux is assessed along with motion of the MTP joint and the location of tenderness. Pain and callus formation under the lesser MTP joint indicates mechanical stress transfer due to incompetent loading of the hallux. Standing radiographs are obtained to assess alignment and length of the first metatarsal relative to the lesser metatarsals (**Fig. 1**). Arthritis of the MTP joint, bony healing, and configuration of any prior osteotomy are also sought. An axial sesamoid radiograph can also assist in determining the presence of subluxation or arthritis.

Malunions are initially treated nonoperatively, focusing on shoewear and orthotic devices. Wide toebox shoes with soft uppers, low heel, and a comfortable fit are

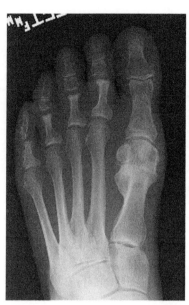

Fig. 1. Anteroposterior radiograph demonstrating shortening after first metatarsal osteotomy.

recommended; fashion footwear is to be avoided. Full-length orthotics are prescribed incorporating a build-up under the hallux to improve its relative weight bearing along with a metatarsal pad to offload the lesser MTP joints and relieve metatarsalgia. A carbon fiber Morton's extension can be added if the hallux MTP joint demonstrates stiffness or arthritic changes.

Surgery is typically considered when appropriate nonoperative attempts have failed an adequate trial (2–3 months). A dorsal cheilectomy can be attempted if the dorsal malunion causes dorsal impingement of the first MTP without severe shortening. If metatarsalgia of the lesser toes coexists, however, a cheilectomy alone would not be effective as it would not address the overload of the lesser toes. A corrective plantar flexion osteotomy of the distal first metatarsal can be performed by either a distal extraarticular crescentic osteotomy from a medial to lateral direction or dorsal opening wedge osteotomy with a bone graft. Such attempted reconstruction can only be attempted if the patient has adequate motion of the first MTP joint. Angular correction or lengthening of the first metatarsal may cause stiffness of the soft tissues surrounding the joint. If the patient has severely limited motion of the MTP joint, then arthrodesis may be a more realistic option. A crescentic osteotomy is indicated if there is little bony shortening, while an opening wedge osteotomy with graft is preferred to restore length. The use of a laminar spreader or distraction device assists in correcting deformity, allowing for intraoperative fluoroscopy to assess the reduction (**Fig. 2**). K-wires are used for provisional fixation while any structural bone graft is fashioned with a saw to fill the defect (**Fig. 3**). After insertion of the graft, fixation consists of screws, pins, or low profile plates. Use of external fixation for a distal malunion can be challenging due to the small distal fragment involved. Hurst and Nunley[22] describe their technique and outcomes for their treatment of five patients with shortened first metatarsals after hallux valgus surgery. They performed first metatarsal lengthening using an external fixator. Mean time to consolidation was 15.8 weeks, with all

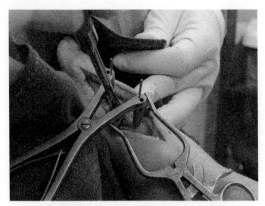

Fig. 2. Intraoperative photo demonstrating use of distraction device to open medial osteotomy site for bone graft wedge insertion.

osteotomies healing. There were no complications and all patients returned to nonantalgic gait Acute lengthening of the first metatarsal is often associated with increased stiffness of the first MTP joint due to soft tissue contracture. Any soft tissue deformity must be addressed, correcting contracture of the MTP capsule or extensor hallucis longus tendon. Osteotomy of the distal first metatarsal can be combined with a shortening osteotomy of the symptomatic lesser metatarsals, particularly if these have excessive length relative to the first metatarsal; clear numeric criteria on the ideal relative lengths, however, remain to be defined and the decision to shorten the lesser metatarsals remains a clinical one.

VARUS/VALGUS MALUNION

Varus or valgus malunions can occur following distal osteotomy with loss of fixation and varus or valgus tilting of the capital fragment (**Fig. 4**). This may also combine a degree of dorsiflexion as well as shortening. Patients with varus or valgus malunions are difficult to treat conservatively due to impingement of the hallux against the shoe toe box or the adjacent toe, respectively. Varus malunion can be treated with a medial opening wedge osteotomy with a bone block graft (**Fig. 5**). Valgus malunion is more

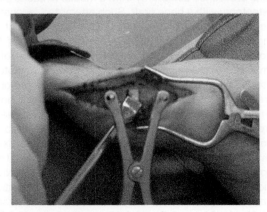

Fig. 3. Insertion of wedge-shaped bone graft into first metatarsal osteotomy site.

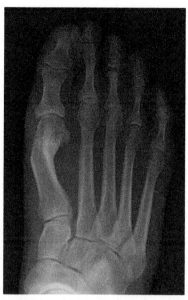

Fig. 4. Anteroposterior radiograph of valgus malunion and shortening of chevron osteotomy. Note tilting of articular surface and incongruity of MTP joint.

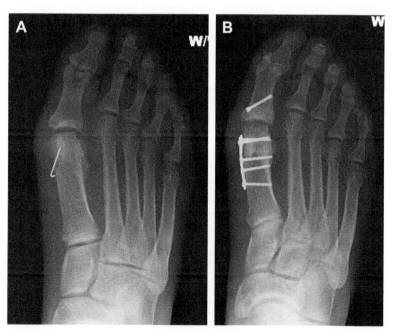

Fig. 5. Anteroposterior radiographs of varus malunion following chevron osteotomy. (*A*) Preoperative view. (*B*) Postoperative view following medial opening wedge osteotomy with bone block graft. Note improved alignment of distal articular surface.

difficult to address, as a medial closing wedge osteotomy can result in further shortening. An alternative method would be a dorsal approach to the distal metatarsal with a lateral opening wedge osteotomy or a crescentic osteotomy. These osteotomies can be fixed with screws and a low profile standard or locking plate. Associated soft tissue deformity must also be corrected, such as medial or lateral joint contracture. Patients with varus or valgus malunion with concomitant arthritis of the first MTP joint are better addressed with MTP arthrodesis, which can alleviate pain and restore alignment in a predictable fashion.

Plantarflexion Malunion

Plantarflexion malunion is very rare with distal osteotomies commonly performed for hallux valgus. Due to the ground reaction force with weight bearing, dorsiflexion malunion is far more common than plantarflexion deformity. A plantarflexion malunion may result from malpositioning intraoperatively or due to catastrophic hardware failure. This can also occur following various metatarsal osteotomies that have been described as joint-sparing alternatives for hallux rigidus (see the article by Seibert and Kadakia in this issue) (**Fig. 6**A). These osteotomies theoretically decompress the first MTP joint and counteract hypothetical metatarsus elevatus by shortening and plantarflexing the metatarsal head. Plantarflexion malunion leads to increased pressure under the first MTP joint, a situation which may be complicated by the presence of joint arthritis. Nonsurgical treatment focuses on a trial of an orthotic insole with a relief under the first MTP joint along with a steel or carbon fiber Morton's extension to reduce bending at the joint. Analgesics, low-impact activity, and judicious use of intraarticular corticosteroid injections may help as well. If these methods fail, surgical treatment attempts to realign the distal fragment with either a dorsal closing wedge osteotomy or a crescentic osteotomy from a medial approach (**Fig. 6**B). This latter method may result in less shortening and better assist in rebalancing forefoot pressures. If the patient has significant arthritic involvement of the MTP joint or the metatarsosesamoid articulation, then MTP fusion provides a more reliable correction and

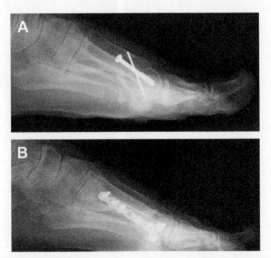

Fig. 6. Lateral radiographs of plantarflexion malunion of distal metatarsal osteotomy. (*A*) Preoperative view. (*B*) Postoperative view following lengthening osteotomy with bone block graft.

better pain relief; in such circumstances, joint-sparing revision surgery may be fraught with complications such as joint stiffness or overcorrection with resultant transfer metatarsalgia.

Rotational Malunion

Rotational malunions of the distal first metatarsal represent complex deformities. Typically due to fixation failure, these deformities can adversely affect the kinematics of the MTP joint, leading to restricted motion, pain, and, ultimately, degenerative arthritis. Attempts at conservative management are rarely successful, as orthotic management cannot adequately correct the deformity and stiffness. Surgical management can consider a derotational osteotomy. This can be a complicated endeavor, as it should combine correction of angulation or shortening as well. Fusion of the MTP joint is certainly warranted if there is evidence of arthritis; it may also prove to be a more predictable and effective option even in the absence of arthritis if the patient has significant stiffness or if three-dimensional deformity correction proves complicated.

PROXIMAL OSTEOTOMY MALUNION

Proximal first metatarsal osteotomies and fractures of the proximal first metatarsal are subject to higher bending moments secondary to the increased lever arm of the first metatarsal shaft. This in turn results in higher rates of malunions, nonunions and loss of fixation. Various osteotomies have been devised for hallux valgus to allow adequate correction of the intermetatarsal angle while trying to optimize technical ease and fixation strength.

The proximal crescentic osteotomy, as popularized by Mann et al.,[23] uses a curved oscillating saw to create a dome-shaped basilar osteotomy. The intermetatarsal angle is corrected by rotating and shifting the distal shaft fragment over the proximal dome. This osteotomy has no intrinsic stability, and tends to fail through fracture of the dorsal bone bridge at the screw head, allowing elevation of the distal fragment.[24] Brodsky and colleagues[25] reported on 32 consecutive proximal crescentic osteotomies at a mean of 29 months follow up. Twelve patients had first metatarsal elevation of greater than 2 mm, with transfer lesions developing in five of these patients.[25] Thordarson and colleagues[26,27] reported their results of 33 proximal crescentic osteotomies. He noted an average dorsiflexion malunion of 6.2° through the osteotomy site, and a varus malalignment in 12% of patients.

The Ludloff osteotomy extends from the dorsal aspect of the proximal metaphysis to the plantar aspect of the diaphysis distally.[28] Despite the lack of inherent stability of the oblique cut, the Ludloff osteotomy has a broad surface for screw fixation, which substantially increases the strength of the construct as described by Acevedo and colleagues.[24] Acevedo also notes that the Ludloff osteotomy resulted in excellent fatigue endurance under cyclic loading. Trnka and colleagues[29,30] report their results of 111 feet treated with Ludloff osteotomies for moderate to severe deformities with an average follow up of 34 months. All osteotomy sites united without any dorsiflexion malunions but with a mean first metatarsal shortening of 2.2 mm.

The scarf osteotomy was introduced by Zygmunt in 1989 and has become increasingly popular in Europe and North America. This z-shaped horizontal osteotomy provides remarkable inherent stability as a result of its long dorsal bony shelf resisting the dorsally directed forces during weight bearing. Jones and colleagues[31] reviewed their results after 35 scarf osteotomies at a mean follow up of 20 months. Excellent radiographic and clinical outcomes were attained with only one intraoperative fracture noted.[31-33] Coetzee,[34] however, report poor results after 20 consecutive scarf osteotomies with high rates of complications. The most common complication in 35% of patients was malunion secondary to troughing of the osteotomy. Troughing occurs when the distal fragment rotates axially as the medial cortex of the distal fragment slides in the medullary canal of the proximal fragment, resulting in elevation and supination of the hallux. In addition, fracture through the thin proximal bony shelf occurred in 10% and delayed union occurred in 5% of patients.

The proximal chevron osteotomy shares the geometric properties and inherent stability of the distal chevron osteotomy. However, the proximal location makes this a more powerful osteotomy and allows correction of more severe deformities. Sammarco and colleagues[35] report their results on 72 consecutive patients treated with a proximal chevron osteotomy and followed for 41 months. They found good clinical results without any dorsal malunion, significant shortening, or new symptoms of metatarsalgia. Markbreiter and Thompson[32] reported results comparing the proximal chevron osteotomy with the proximal crescentic osteotomy in 50 feet. Both had good clinical outcomes, but the chevron osteotomy was thought to be technically easier to perform because of its inherent stability. A medial proximal opening wedge osteotomy combined with a distal soft tissue procedure is also an option for correction of moderate hallux valgus deformities. Cooper and colleagues[36] published their technique and outcomes with plate fixation for medial opening wedge osteotomy. Their results show two (8.6%) valgus malunions and one (4%) delayed union.

Complications following proximal osteotomies or fractures of the first metatarsal are not uncommon. One of the most common postoperative complications is a dorsal malunion (**Fig. 7**). A dorsal malunion with shortening of the first metatarsal usually presents with complaints of transfer lesions secondary to overload of the lesser toes. This can be treated with a full-length orthotic with a build-up beneath the distal first metatarsal. If a patient fails orthotic treatment and use of appropriate footwear, this problem can be treated with a dorsal opening wedge osteotomy. A dorsal opening wedge osteotomy plantarflexes as well as restores length to the first metatarsal using a bony autologous or allograft wedge. An alternative option would be a crescentic osteotomy created from the medial side. The distal fragment is then rotated and plantarflexed. Fixation with either technique consists of low profile plates and screws. If the bone quality is poor and adequate fixation is a concern, or if there is instability with a hypermobile first ray, dorsal malunion can be treated with a Lapidus fusion (first tarsometatarsal arthrodesis). The arthrodesis site preparation includes additional resection plantarly or a plantar wedge resection to allow relative plantarflexion of

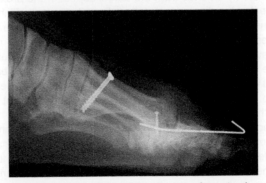

Fig. 7. Lateral radiograph showing dorsiflexion malunion of proximal crescentic osteotomy. Note elevation of first metatarsal relative to remaining metatarsals.

the metatarsal to reestablish weight bearing function. Coetzee and colleagues[37,38] describe using the Lapidus procedure for salvage after a failed osteotomy with good results. However, he warns that the downside of using this procedure may lead to additional shortening of the metatarsal and transfer overload of the lesser metatarsals. The presence of preexisting transfer metatarsalgia would suggest the need for concomitant lesser metatarsal-shortening osteotomy.

FIRST METATARSAL NONUNION

Nonunions of first metatarsal osteotomies or fractures are relatively rare (**Fig. 8**). Most distal and proximal osteotomies are performed in either the metaphyseal portion of the metatarsal, with primarily cancellous bone, or longitudinally in the diaphysis with long surface area for healing. The literature on the nonunion rates of fractures or osteotomies of the first metatarsal is sparse. Theoretically, nonunions may have been more common before contemporary internal fixation methods were broadly adopted. Proximal osteotomies and fractures may have higher rates of nonunion due to the increased mechanical stress from the longer lever arm as previously discussed.

Although rarely encountered, nonunions are usually symptomatic, presenting with pain, transfer metatarsalgia, and stiffness of the first MTP joint. Initial management efforts can focus on analgesia, avoidance of high-impact or exacerbating activities, and comfortable footwear. A full-length orthotic insole with a Morton's extension can be prescribed to splint and protect the nonunion site. The treatment of nonunions and stress fractures of the metatarsals with external electrical stimulation and ultrasound therapy has been successful in recent studies. Holmes and colleagues published their experience with treatment of fifth metatarsal nonunions with pulsed electrical magnetic field (PEMF). Nine nonunions treated with PEMF all healed in a mean time of 4 months.[39] Nolte and colleagues[40] published his results of treating established nonunions of long bones including metatarsal fractures. With 20 minutes of low intensity ultrasound therapy daily, 86% of fractures healed in a mean time of 22 weeks. Direct applicability to nonunions of the first metatarsal, however, remains ill-defined. The overall success rate of nonsurgical treatment for first metatarsal nonunion is not known.

Revision surgery is indicated if the patient remains symptomatic despite attempted conservative treatment. Evidence of progressive deformity or instability of the nonunion site also necessitates surgery. The quality of bone stock and degree of deformity dictate the surgical options. In cases with good bone stock, debridement and drilling of the nonunion site is followed by bone grafting and rigid internal fixation with lag screws or plates/screw constructs. If the nonunion site has avascular bone or if there is excessive shortening secondary to bone loss, debridement of the necrotic

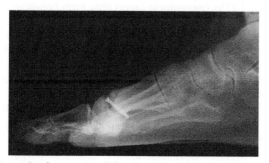

Fig. 8. Lateral radiograph of nonunion following distal chevron osteotomy.

segments and use of structural autologous or allograft bone block lengthening with rigid internal fixation is recommended. Nonunion associated with deformity is addressed by debridement, bone grafting, deformity correction, and fixation. Correction of such deformity is analogous to the description of surgery for first metatarsal malunion.

AVASCULAR NECROSIS OF THE FIRST METATARSAL

Avascular necrosis or osteonecrosis of the first metatarsal head is very rare. This occurs most often following corrective surgery for hallux valgus, in particular a distal metatarsal osteotomy with a lateral soft tissue release or significant distal soft tissue stripping. Spontaneous causes have also been described including trauma, corticosteroid use, vasculitis, hemoglobinopathies, and alcoholism.[41] Easley and colleagues[42–44] describe the first ray as having a significant capacity to withstand and compensate for a vascular insult until there is joint involvement and collapse.

The vascular anatomy of the first metatarsal is complex. The blood supply includes the nutrient artery, the periosteal capillary network, and the metaphyseal capsular vessels. All of these vessels are branches of the first dorsal metatarsal artery, which originates from the dorsalis pedis artery. The dorsal vessels supply two thirds of the head while the plantar vessels supply the remaining third. Distal osteotomies disrupt the intraosseous blood supply, as they are typically performed distal to the penetration point of the nutrient artery. This leaves the capsular vessels as the only remaining blood supply, which can easily be disrupted with excessive lateral soft tissue stripping or overpenetration by the saw blade while creating an osteotomy. Historically, the incidence of AVN has been reported as high as 72%. Meier and Kenzora[45] reported AVN rates following a chevron osteotomy alone of 20%, and 40% when combined with a lateral soft tissue release. Subsequent literature, however, has questioned this high incidence.[46–48] Trnka and colleagues[38] observed three cases of AVN out of 94 when a distal osteotomy was combined with a lateral soft tissue release through a first webspace incision. Vora and Myerson[46] comment on their results of 1430 chevron osteotomies performed with only two incidences of AVN. In addition Jones and colleagues[49] published results of chevron osteotomies performed with lateral soft tissue releases with only a 2% incidence of AVN, showing that careful handling of soft tissue with minimal stripping is safe during the lateral release. Kuhn and colleagues[21,50] describe the vascular insult to the blood supply of the first metatarsal head after a chevron osteotomy and lateral soft tissue release using a Doppler probe to monitor blood flow. They show the greatest insult occurred following medial capsulotomy, with a 45% decrease in blood flow. The lateral release caused a 13% decrease and the chevron osteotomy itself caused an additional 13% decrease. They observed a total 71% decrease in blood flow from baseline, yet there were no cases of AVN in their 20 consecutive patients.[50] It is now generally accepted that the risk of AVN following distal metatarsal osteotomy combined with lateral capsular release is very low with meticulous surgical technique and if excessive soft tissue stripping is avoided.

Patient presentations and symptoms vary greatly, with many patients essentially asymptomatic. The radiographic findings and symptoms may not coincide with the level of symptoms. Patients may demonstrate pain and swelling of the MTP joint, stiffness, and transfer metatarsalgia secondary to collapse and shortening of the first ray in advanced cases. A continuum of radiographic findings occur with AVN, including subchondral lucencies and focal cysts (**Fig. 9**), bony collapse, fragmentation and joint space narrowing with advanced arthritis. MRI is a very specific examination for the

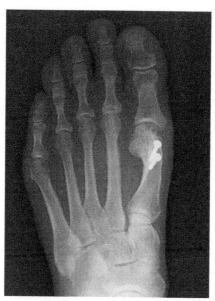

Fig. 9. Anteroposterior radiograph demonstrating early avascular necrosis of first metatarsal head. Note lucencies and cystic changes.

diagnosis of AVN, and can show the extent of head involvement. MRI findings suggestive of AVN are decreased signal intensity on T1 and increased signal intensity on T2.

The management of patients with AVN depends on the degree of symptoms and extent of disease involvement. Because most patients are asymptomatic or present with mild pain and stiffness, they can be initially managed nonoperatively. This would

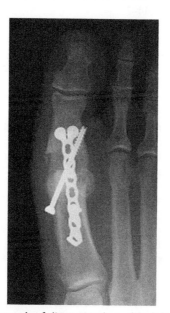

Fig. 10. Anteroposterior radiograph of distraction bone block first MTP arthrodesis.

include a stiff-soled shoe or an orthotic insole with a Morton's extension to decrease the motion and repetitive stress experienced by the first MTP joint. In patients with more severe pain and swelling along with moderate joint involvement, good results with joint debridement and subchondral drilling of the metatarsal head have been reported by Fu and colleagues.[43] Arthrodesis of the first MTP joint is indicated if there is significant joint space narrowing, arthritis, or metatarsal head collapse. Extra care needs to be taken during preparation of the joint as the metatarsal head is brittle and may fragment easily. If there is shortening of the first metatarsal as a result of bone collapse or if a segment of bone needs to be resected to provide a viable bony interface for fusion, a distraction bone block arthrodesis should be performed to restore the length of the first ray (**Fig. 10**).[51]

REFERENCES

1. Veri JP, Pirani SP, Claridge R. Crescentic proximal metatarsal osteotomy for moderate to severe hallux valgus; a mean of 12.2 year follow up study. Foot Ankle Int 2001;22:817–22.
2. Shereff MJ, Sobel MA, Kummer FJ. The stability of fixation of first metatarsal osteotomies. Foot Ankle Int 1991;11:208–11.
3. Austin DW, Leventen EO. A new osteotomy for hallux valgus; a horizontally directed V displacement osteotomy of the metatarsal head for hallux valgus and primus varus. Clin Orthop Rel Res 1981;157:25–30.
4. Sammarco VJ. Surgical correction of moderate and severe hallux valgus; proximal metatarsal osteotomy with distal soft tissue correction and arthrodesis of the metatarsophalangeal joint. J Bone Joint Surg Am 2007;89:2520–31.
5. Thompson FM. Complications of hallux valgus surgery and salvage. Orthopedics 1990;13(9):1059–67.
6. Johnson KA, Cofield RH, Morrey BF. Chevron osteotomy for hallux valgus. Clin Orthop Rel Res 1979;142:44–7.
7. Trnka HJ, Zembsch A, Easely M, et al. The chevron osteotomy for correction of hallux valgus: comparison of findings after 2 and 5 years of follow up. J Bone Joint Surg Am 2000;82:1373–8.
8. Mitchell CL, Fleming JL, Allen R, et al. Osteotomy-bunionectomy for hallux valgus. J Bone Joint Surg Am 1958;40:41–58.
9. Trnka H, Zembsch A, Weisauer H, et al. Modified Austin procedure for correction of hallux valgus. Foot Ankle Int 1997;19:119–27.
10. Lian GJ, Markoff K, Cracchiolo A. Strength of fixation constructs for basilar osteotomies of the first metatarsal. Foot Ankle 1992;13:509–14.
11. Teli M, Grassi FA, Montolli C, et al. The Mitchell bunionectomy; a prospective study of 60 consecutive cases utilizing single k-wire fixation. J Foot Ankle Surg 2001;40:144–51.
12. Gill LH. Distal osteotomy for bunionectomy and hallux valgus correction. Foot Ankle Clin 2001;6:433–53.
13. Myerson MS. Reconstructive foot and ankle surgery. Philadelphia: Elsevier Saunders; 2005. p. 61–8.
14. Scioli MW. Complications of hallux valgus surgery and subsequent treatment options. Foot Ankle Clin 1997;2:719–39.
15. Shereff MJ, Ynag QM, Kummer FJ. Extraosseous and intraosseous arterial supply to the first metatarsal and metatarsophalangeal joint. Foot Ankle 1987; 8:81–93.

16. Fokter SK, Podobnik J, Vengust V. Late results of modified Mitchell procedure for the treatment of hallux valgus. Foot Ankle Int 1999;20:296–300.

17. Jahss MH, Troy AI, Kummer F. Roentgenographic and mathematical analysis of first metatarsal osteotomies for metatarsus primus valgus: a comparative study. Foot Ankle 1985;5:280–321.

18. Saro C, Andren B, Wildemyr Z, et al. Outcome after distal metatarsal osteotomy for hallux valgus; a prospective randomized controlled trial of two methods. J Bone Joint Surg Am 2007;28:778–87.

19. Bosch P, Wenke S, Lengstein R. Hallux valgus correction by the method of Bosch: a new technique with seven to ten year follow up. Foot Ankle Clin 2000;5(3): 485–98.

20. Portaluri M. Hallux valgus correction by method of Bosch: a clinical evaluation. Foot Ankle Clin 2000;5(3):499–511.

21. Kadakia AR, Smerek JP, Myerson MS. Radiographic results after percutaneous distal metatarsal osteotomy for correction of hallux valgus deformity. Foot Ankle Int 2007;28:355–60.

22. Hurst JM, Nunley JA. Distraction osteogenesis for the shortened metatarsal after hallux valgus surgery. Foot Ankle Int 2007;28(2):194–8.

23. Mann RA, Rudicel S, Graves SC. Repair of hallux valgus with distal soft tissue procedure and proximal metatarsal osteotomy. J Bone Joint Surg Am 1992;7: 124–9.

24. Acevedo JI, Sammarco J, Boucher HR, et al. Mechanical comparison of cyclic loading in five different first metatarsal shaft osteotomies. Foot Ankle Int 2002; 23:711–6.

25. Brodsky JW, Beischer AD, Robinson AH, et al. Surgery for hallux valgus with proximal crescentic osteotomy causes variable postoperative pressure patterns. Clin Orthop Rel Res 2006;443:280–6.

26. Thordarson DB, Leventen EO. Hallux valgus correction with proximal metatarsal osteotomy: two year follow up. Foot Ankle Int 1992;13:321–6.

27. Stokes AF, Hutton WC, Stott JRR. Forces acting on the metatarsal during normal walking. J Anat 1979;129:579–90.

28. Chiodo CP, Schon LC, Myerson MS. Clinical results with the Ludloff metatarsal osteotomy for correction of adult hallux valgus. Foot Ankle Int 2004;25:532–6.

29. Trnka HJ. Osteotomies for hallux valgus correction. Foot Ankle Clin 2005;10: 15–33.

30. Lehman DE. Salvage of complications of hallux valgus surgery. Foot Ankle Clin 2003;8:15–35.

31. Jones S, Al Hussainy HA, Ali F, et al. Scarf osteotomy for hallux valgus. A prospective clinical and pedobarographic study. J Bone Joint Surg Br 2004;86: 830–6.

32. Markbreiter LA, Thompson FM. Proximal metatarsal osteotomy in hallux valgus correction: a comparison of crescentic and chevron procedures. Foot Ankle Int 1997;18:71–6.

33. Grimes JS, Coughlin MJ. First metatarsophalangeal joint arthrodesis as a treatment for failed hallux valgus surgery. Foot Ankle Int 2006;27:887–93.

34. Coetzee JC. Scarf osteotomy for hallux valgus repair; the dark side. Foot Ankle Int 2003;24:29–33.

35. Sammarco GJ, Brainard BJ, Sammarco VJ. Bunion correction using proximal chevron osteotomy. Foot Ankle 1983;14:8–14.

36. Cooper MT, Berlet GC, Shurnas PS, et al. Proximal opening wedge osteotomy of the first metatarsal for correction of hallux valgus. Surg Technol Int 2007;16:215–9.

37. Coetzee JC, Resig S, Kuskowski M, et al. The Lapidus procedure as salvage after failed surgical treatment of hallux valgus. J Bone Joint Surg Am 2003;85:60–5.
38. Trnka HJ, Parks B, Ivanic G, et al. Six first metatarsal shaft osteotomies: mechanical and immobilization comparisons. Clin Orthop Rel Res 2000;381:256–65.
39. GB Holmes. Treatment of delayed unions and nonunions of the proximal fifth metatarsal with pulsed electromagnetic fields. Foot Ankle Int 1994;15(10):552–6.
40. Nolte PA, van der Krans P, Patka P, et al. Low intensity pulsed ultrasound in the treatment of nonunions. J Trauma 2001;51(4):702–3.
41. Banks AS. Avascular necrosis of the first metatarsal head. J Am Podiatr Med Assoc 1999;89(9):441–53.
42. Easley ME, Kelly IP. Avascular necrosis of the hallux metatarsal head. Foot Ankle Clin 2000;5(3):591–608.
43. Fu FH, Gomez W. Bilateral avascular necrosis of the first metatarsal in adolescence. A case report. Clin Orthop Rel Res 1988;246:282–4.
44. Brodsky JW, Ptaszek AJ, Morris SG. Salvage first MTP arthrodesis utilizing ICBG: clinical evaluation and outcome. Foot Ankle Int 2000;21:290–6.
45. Meier PJ, Kenzora JE. The risks and benefits of distal first metatarsal osteotomies. Foot Ankle 1985;6(1):7–17.
46. Vora AM, Myerson MS. First metatarsal osteotomy nonunion and malunion. Foot Ankle Clin 2005;10:35–54.
47. Sammarco VJ, Acevedo J. Stability and fixation techniques in first metatarsal osteotomies. Foot Ankle Clin 2001;6:409–32.
48. Easely ME, Kiezvbak GM, Davis WH, et al. Prospective randomized comparison of proximal crescentic and proximal chevron osteotomies for correction of hallux valgus deformity. Foot Ankle Int 1996;17:307–16.
49. Jones KJ, Feiwell LA, Freedman EL. The effect of chevron osteotomy with lateral capsular release on the blood supply to the first metatarsal head. J Bone Joint Surg Am 1995;77:197.
50. Kuhn MA, Lippert FG, Phipps MJ, et al. Blood flow to the metatarsal head after chevron bunionectomy. Foot Ankle Int 2005;26:526–9.
51. Myerson MS, Schon LC, McGuigan FX, et al. Result of arthrodesis of the hallux metatarsophalangeal joint using bone graft for restoration of length. Foot Ankle Int 2000;21:297–306.

Hallux Sesamoid Disorders

Bruce E. Cohen, MD

KEYWORDS

- Sesamoid • Hallux • Sesamoiditis • Osteochondrosis
- Osteonecrosis • Stress fracture

The hallucal sesamoids are two seed-shaped bones that form an integral portion of the hallux metatarsophalangeal joint complex. The sesamoids function to absorb weight-bearing forces, decrease friction, and protect the flexor hallucis brevis tendons. The sesamoids increase the moment of the flexor hallucis brevis, which powers plantar flexion of the hallux. A final function of the hallucal sesamoids is to elevate the first metatarsal head, which functions to dissipate the forces on the metatarsal head.[1–4] Disorders that affect the sesamoid complex can compromise function of the hallux metatarsophalangeal complex. Because of the significant mechanical stresses and anatomic variations, the sesamoid complex appears to be involved in numerous pathologic processes. These processes include acute fractures, stress fractures, nonunions, osteonecrosis, chondromalacia, and various inflammatory conditions labeled sesamoiditis.

The sesamoids typically ossify by the age of 8 years in girls and 12 years in boys.[2] The sesamoids can develop in partitioned fashion. Termed bipartite or multipartite, such incomplete fusion more commonly involves the tibial sesamoid with an incidence of 10% and a chance of bilaterality of 25%. A bipartite fibular sesamoid is rare.[3] The medial, or tibial, sesamoid is the larger of the two, which effectively increases its impact on weight bearing and therefore its propensity for injury. Both sesamoids are embedded in the tendons of the flexor hallucis brevis.[3] The sesamoids are held together by the intersesamoid ligament. The tibial sesamoid is tethered by the abductor hallucis and the medial portion of the flexor hallucis brevis, whereas the oblique and transverse heads of the abductor hallucis muscle attach to the fibular sesamoid.[2] Additional attachments include the medial sesamoid ligament, which courses from the metatarsal head to the medial aspect of the tibial sesamoid, and the lateral sesamoidal ligament, which runs from the metatarsal head to the fibular sesamoid. These two structures and the thick intersesamoidal ligament come together to attach to the plantar plate. The intermetatarsal ligament attaches the fibular sesamoid to the second metatarsal neck (**Fig. 1**A and B).[1]

OrthoCarolina Foot and Ankle Institute, 1001 Blythe Boulevard, Suite 200, Charlotte, NC 28203, USA
E-mail address: bruce.cohen@orthocarolina.com

Foot Ankle Clin N Am 14 (2009) 91–104
doi:10.1016/j.fcl.2008.11.003

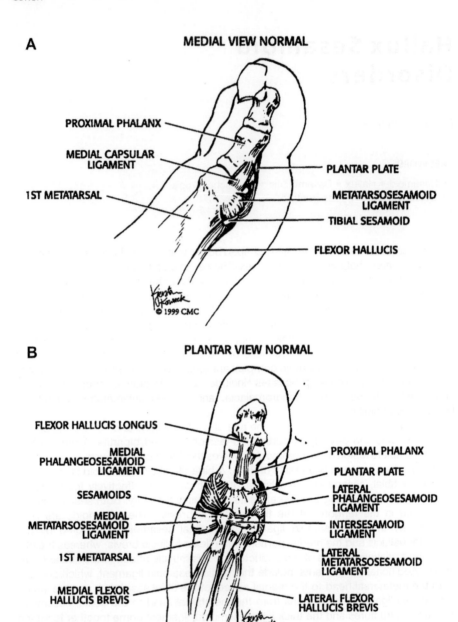

A

MEDIAL VIEW NORMAL

PROXIMAL PHALANX

MEDIAL CAPSULAR LIGAMENT

1ST METATARSAL

PLANTAR PLATE

METATARSOSESAMOID LIGAMENT

TIBIAL SESAMOID

FLEXOR HALLUCIS

© 1999 CMC

B

PLANTAR VIEW NORMAL

FLEXOR HALLUCIS LONGUS

MEDIAL PHALANGEOSESAMOID LIGAMENT

SESAMOIDS

MEDIAL METATARSOSESAMOID LIGAMENT

1ST METATARSAL

MEDIAL FLEXOR HALLUCIS BREVIS

PROXIMAL PHALANX

PLANTAR PLATE

LATERAL PHALANGEOSESAMOID LIGAMENT

INTERSESAMOID LIGAMENT

LATERAL METATARSOSESAMOID LIGAMENT

LATERAL FLEXOR HALLUCIS BREVIS

© 1999 CMC

Fig. 1. (*A*) Medial view of hallux metatarsal phalangeal joint. (*B*) Plantar view of hallux metatarsal phalangeal joint. (*Courtesy of* the Carolinas Medical Center, Charlotte, NC; with permission.)

BLOOD SUPPLY

The osseous blood supply to the sesamoids is complex and has been found to be primarily extraosseous. The major blood supply arises from the proximal and plantar direction. The tibial and fibular sesamoid receives equal vascularity.[5] The plantar vascular supply is provided by the proper plantar artery and the first plantar metatarsal artery. The first plantar metatarsal artery arises from either the plantar arch (25%), the medial plantar artery (25%), or both (50%).[1] The distal blood supply is via the synovial capsule and is relatively low volume. It should be noted that the distal vascular supply is more dorsal and the only intraosseous blood supply is from proximal to dorsal.[6] Because of the predominately plantar vascular supply, plantar surgical approaches and blunt plantar trauma can compromise circulation. The safest interval for surgical approaches is the medial approach.[7]

CLINICAL EVALUATION

It is important to localize the pain when evaluating the metatarsal sesamoid complex. The patients can have an acute presentation from a specific traumatic event. Pain is often of insidious onset and typically presents unilaterally. Pain with weight bearing is the most common complaint and certain shoe wear can exacerbate symptoms. Because the tibial sesamoid is more often symptomatic, the pain is typically located medially and plantarly. For the fibular sesamoid involvement, the pain is plantar lateral. Passive range of motion of the hallux metatarsalphalangeal (MTP) joint may be pain-less. Direct tenderness and tenderness on resisted plantar flexion of the hallux are classic signs of sesamoid pathology. The presence of an enlarged bursa on the plantar surface is not uncommon. Attention to mechanical alignment of the foot is important because malposition may lead to increased plantar pressure on the sesamoids.Significant pes cavus or planus can cause alteration of the weight-bearing forces on the MTP joint, as can significant hallux valgus or varus. With instances of instability of the hallux MTP joint from disruption of the plantar soft tissues, an abnormal sagittal plane translation may be present such as cocking up of the toe.

RADIOLOGY

Radiographic evaluation of sesamoid disorders is an integral part of the examination. Various factors need to be taken into account in determining both the etiology of the deformity as well as the treatment options. Standard radiographs include weight-bearing anteroposterior, oblique, and lateral views as well as an axial sesamoid view. This axial sesamoid view is a tangential view of the sesamoids and lesser meta-tarsal heads obtained by directing the beam at the forefoot in a tangential manner while the forefoot is in a dorsiflexed position (**Fig. 2**).[8] This view can indicate malalign-ment relative to the metatarsal head as well as identify the presence of arthritis

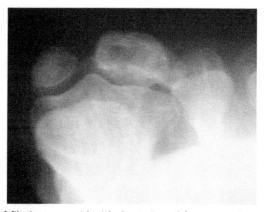

Fig. 2. Axial view of fibular sesamoid with diastasis and fragmentation.

between the sesamoids and the metatarsal. Pertinent findings on plain radiography include acute fractures, presence of bipartite or multipartite sesamoid, signs of osteonecrosis, hallux MTP alignment, and sesamoid location (proximal retraction, diastasis, or medial or lateral translation).

Differentiating between a partitioned or bipartite sesamoid and a fractured sesamoid can be accomplished using standard radiographs. Bilaterality is a hallmark of a partitioned sesamoid, whereas bilateral fractures are extremely rare. When present bilaterally, a partitioned sesamoid is symmetric in location approximately 84% of the time (**Fig. 3**). A fractured sesamoid is characterized by an irregular pattern, the presence of sharp fracture edges, comminution, or wide separation and diastasis of fragments.[9]

Other pathologic entities have characteristic radiographic features as well. Osteonecrosis is characterized by radiolucency, sclerosis of fragments, and, in later stages, fragmentation.[9] Infection has the findings of focal osteoporosis, cortical disruption, separation of fragments, and, less frequently, periostitis of adjacent metatarsals.[9]

Radionuclide or skeletal scintigraphy has historically been used to assist in the diagnosis of sesamoid disorders. If the diagnosis is unclear, a technetium bone scan can assist in localizing the region of pathology indicated by increased uptake of radionuclide tracer (**Fig. 4**A,B). Magnetic resonance imaging (MRI) is a more specific modality to diagnose sesamoid disorders. MRI scanning allows differentiation between osseous abnormalities and soft tissue pathology. The best plane for MRI evaluation is the coronal plane, perpendicular to the long axis of the metatarsal. The next most useful series of images is the sagittal series, whereas axial plane views are less helpful. The techniques used include T1 images, which highlight fat, and T2 images, which highlight edema. Within the T2 images it is helpful to obtain fat suppression or STIR, short inversion time interval, images to improve sensitivity of identifying bony edema (**Fig. 5**A,B).

The following entities have characteristic MRI findings:

Ischemia—always detectable on MRI; more common involving the fibular sesamoid; low signal on T1 and high T2 and STIR images in variable intensities.

Fractures—fracture line seen on sagittal images; low intensity on T1.

Stress Fractures—marrow edema is seen and can replace the normal marrow signal completely; only slight decreased T1 intensity.

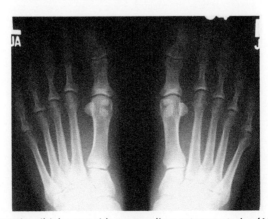

Fig. 3. Bilateral bipartite tibial sesamoids on standing anteroposterior (AP) view.

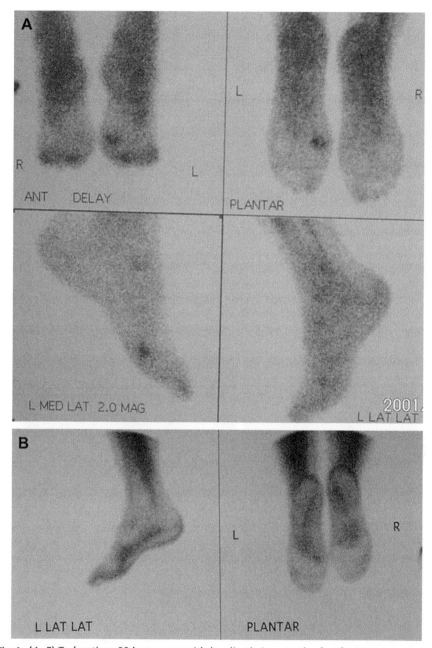

Fig. 4. (*A, B*) Technetium 99 bone scan with localized views to the forefoot.

Sesamoiditis—the standard radiographs are unremarkable; contrast may help differentiate from osteonecrosis; there is subtle soft tissue involvement seen.
Infection—once again contrast may be helpful when infection is suspected; low T1 signal; high T2 and STIR images.[10]

CT scans are helpful to assess arthritis, acute fractures, or nonunions.

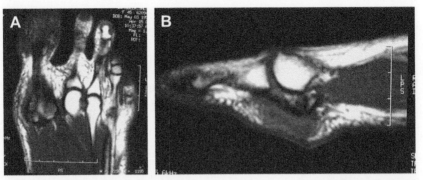

Fig. 5. (*A*) Axial MRI view of tibial sesamoid with avascular necrosis (AVN) and fragmentation. (*B*) Sagittal MRI view of tibial sesamoid with AVN and fragmentation.

SESAMOID FRACTURE

Acute sesamoid fracture can result from direct trauma or a crush injury. Severe trauma can cause complete disruption of the plantar soft tissue restraints and lead to dislocation (**Fig. 6**A,B). The mechanism of an acute fracture is typically forced dorsiflexion. Acute fractures more commonly involve the tibial sesamoid. The fracture appears as a transverse fracture line with sharp, irregular edges. This is in contrast to a nonunion, which is characterized by sclerotic edges and can have evidence of

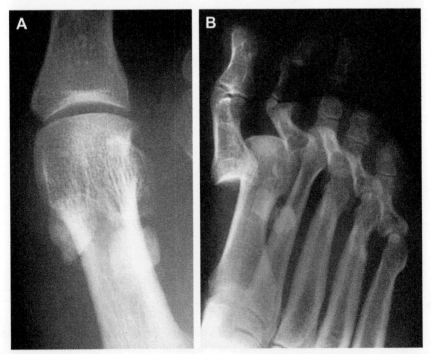

Fig. 6. (*A*) AP view of dislocation of hallux metarsalphalangeal (MP) joint with proximal retraction/position of sesamoids and associated fibular sesamoid fracture with diastasis. (*B*) Oblique view of dislocation of hallux MP joint with proximal retraction/position of sesamoids and associated fibular sesamoid fracture with diastasis.

avascular changes. The treatment of the acute fractures is usually non–weight bearing in a cast with a toe plate for 6 weeks followed by walker boot for 4 to 6 more weeks. Open reduction and internal fixation of acute fractures is controversial and typically reserved for widely displaced fractures.

The diagnosis of a sesamoid stress fracture is suggested by clinical symptoms. It typically is the result of an alteration in normal activity level or increased training intensity by an athlete. The common symptoms are activity-related plantar hallux pain sometimes associated with swelling. Plain radiographs taken early in the disease process are typically normal. MRI scans or technetium bone scan can show abnormal findings before any plain radiographic changes.

The initial treatment of sesamoid nonunion or chronic stress fracture is nonoperative, including rest, activity limitation, and often a period of immobilization. The use of an orthotic designed to off-load the sesamoids and restrict excessive dorsiflexion is essential in nonoperative care. If these measures fail after a period of several months, then operative treatment is considered. There are several surgical options including partial excision of the proximal pole of the sesamoid, complete sesamoidectomy, and bone grafting of the nonunited sesamoid fracture. Biedert and Hinterman[11,12] reported on five athletes with sesamoid fractures treated with excision of the proximal pole of the tibial sesamoid for nonhealing stress fractures while retaining the distal pole. All patients returned to athletics within 6 months of surgical treatment (**Fig. 7**A,B).

McBryde and Anderson[13] described autogenous bone grafting as an alternative to excision. This is performed via a 5-cm plantarmedial incision. Care must be taken to avoid injury to the plantar digital nerve to the hallux. The joint is entered through a medial capsulotomy above the level of the tibial sesamoid. The sesamoid articular surface is inspected as well as the reciprocal surface on the metatarsal head. The capsulotomy is then closed and the sesamiod nonunion is approached through an extraarticular manner. The nonunion is debrided and autogenous bone graft, from the medial eminence of the metatarsal head, is inserted into the defect. The patient is immobilized in a toe-spica cast non–weight bearing for 3 to 4 weeks then transitioned into a weight-bearing cast for approximately 4 weeks. At 8 weeks, active range of motion and gentle passive range of motion is begun. The authors reported on 21 patients and 19 of these active patients went on to union and return to full activity (**Fig. 8**).

INTRACTABLE PLANTAR KERATOSIS

Excessive plantar prominence of the hallux metatarsal phalangeal joint can result in the formation of a painful plantar callosity or intractable plantar keratosis. Mechanical factors that can contribute to this are relative plantarflexion of the first metatarsal, pes cavus, ankle equinus, and stiffness of the metatarsocuneiform joint. A major etiologic factor is iatrogenic causes seen after forefoot procedures. Excessive plantar translation of the first metatarsal with a proximal osteotomy, excessive dorsiflexion of the second metatarsal, excision of one sesamoid, or a previous sesamoid shaving procedure on the adjacent sesamoid are some of the iatrogenic causes.

The clinical presentation is pain located plantarly over the involved sesamoid with a painful localized callosity in this region. The pain is typically with weight bearing and can be temporarily relieved with orthotic management and paring of the hyperkeratosis. It is common for the callosity and symptoms to be recalcitrant to this treatment long term and require surgical management (**Fig. 9**A,B). Sesamoid shaving was originally described by Mann in 1992.[8] The procedure is performed through a medial or

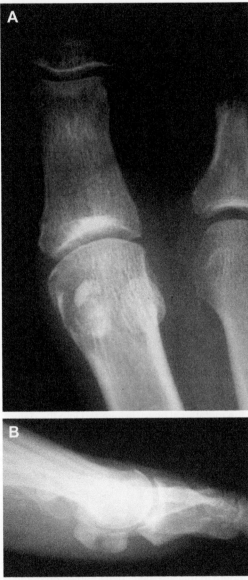

Fig. 7. (*A*) AP radiograph of stress fracture of tibial sesamoid with diastasis. (*B*) Lateral radiograph of stress fracture of tibial sesamoid with diastasis.

plantar incision for the tibial and fibular sesamoids respectively. With care taken to protect the plantar nerves, the sesamoid is thinned from the plantar surface using a microsaggital saw. The amount removed can range from 25% to 50% of the thickness of the sesamoid. Care must be taken to avoid over-resection, which can lead to transfer lesions or even insufficiency fractures of the sesamoid. Additional surgical procedures may be considered to correct an underlying mechanical deformity, such as first metatarsal dorsiflexion osteotomy, pes cavus reconstruction, or gastrocnemius recession or tendoachilles lengthening.

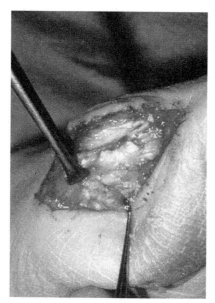

Fig. 8. Curettage and subsequent placement of autogenous bone graft in sesamoid nonunion.

SESAMOIDITIS

Sesamoiditis is a generic term for numerous conditions involving the sesamoids, including osteonecrosis, chondromalacia, or mechanical overload. This can be characterized by avascular changes of the sesamoids or just inflammation of the sesamoid without radiographic changes, fragmentation, fracture, or sclerosis. Patients can also present with a painful swollen plantar bursitis. The etiology is typically repetitive trauma more commonly seen in young adults. Other factors include significant mechanical overload caused by pes cavus, significant plantar flexed first ray, and ankle equinus.[1] Scranton[14] described three variations in the sesamoid anatomy that lead to mechanical overload. These factors include (1) an absent crista, (2) variations in sesamoid size, and (3) significant metatarsal rotation. Avascular necrosis of the

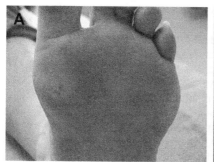
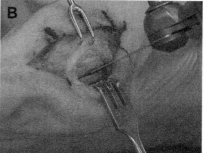

Fig. 9. (A) Clinical photograph of intractable plantar keratosis from tibial sesamoid. (B) Operative photograph demonstrating technique of sesamoid shaving. A saw is used to resect a portion of prominent sesamoid plantar surface.

sesamoids was first described by Ilfeld and Rosen in 1972.[1,8] The description included the early stages, which are characterized by radiographic signs of fragmentation, irregularity, and cystic formation. The later stages classically have sclerosis, collapse, and flattening of the sesamoids.[9] The plain radiographs are characteristic and further diagnosis is confirmed by MRI. Unfortunately, technetium bone scans may have false negatives even with the use of pinhole images.

CONSERVATIVE TREATMENT

Nonoperative treatment is usually the first line of treatment for chronic sesamoid disorders. For acute inflammatory disorders of significant intensity and any fracture/dislocation or severe soft tissue injury, the initial period of immobilization is essential. This immobilization can range from strict non–weight bearing in a toe spica short-leg cast to protected walking in a removable boot orthosis. Orthotic management is essential in off-loading the hallux metatarsal phalangeal complex. In a lower demand patient a metatarsal bar will suffice. The lower profile devices such as a dancer's pad or a transferable metatarsal pad can provide some mechanical relief. Ultimately, a custom-molded orthotic device with elevation proximally and a relief well or visco-elastic polymer under the sesamoids can be very effective. This can be combined with a metal shank or carbon-fiber forefoot plate to restrict forefoot motion and eliminate loading in the dorsiflexed position. The use of nonsteroidal anti-inflammatory medications can be beneficial. Intra-articular corticosteroid injections can be considered on a very limited basis, repeated intra-articular injections should be avoided.

SESAMOIDECTOMY

Surgical excision (sesamoidectomy) is the most common surgical procedure used for treatment of sesamoid pathology. Before considering removal of one or both of the sesamoids it is important to recall their function. They serve to protect the flexor hallucis longus tendon, help transmit load to the medial forefoot, and minimize the joint forces on the first MTP joint by increasing the distance of the flexors from the joint. This function also serves to increase the moment arm and subsequently increase the force genenrated.[15] Several studies by Aper and colleagues[15,16] looked at the effect of various resections of the sesamoids and the effect on the moment arm of the flexor hallucis longus (FHL) and the flexor hallucis brevis. Resection of both sesamoids significantly affected the moment arm of both tendons, whereas all other situations affected only the moment arm of the FHL. Hemiresection or partial excision did not appear to affect the joint mechanics.[15] Therefore, surgical excision of both sesamoids can lead to significant alteration of joint mechanics as well as lead to a cock-up deformity of the hallux because of the loss of plantar restraints.

Sesamoidectomy may be recommended after failure of conservative management for various pathologic entities including fractures, nonunion, osteonecrosis, chondromalacia, and inflammatory disorders. Sesamoidectomy was reported by Mann and colleagues[17–19] to have significant morbidity. In 21 patients, with 13 tibial sesamoidectomies, 50% had continued pain, 60% with plantar flexion weakness, 33% with loss of range of motion, and only 5% with altered hallux alignment. More contemporary series have demonstrated more optimistic outcomes. Brodsky[20] reported a series of sesamoidectomies for fracture, noting that only 2 of 23 patients had postoperative weakness of plantar-flexion. In a recent report, Lee and colleagues[21] reported on 32 patients who underwent tibial sesamoidectomy, with 90% returning to normal activities and demonstrating no significant change in the intermetatarsal angle, hallux valgus angle, or sesamoid station after this procedure. The pedobarographic data demonstrated no evidence of altered plantar pressures in the region of the hallux metatarsal phalangeal joint. Isokinetic measurements of ankle plantar flexion push-off strength did not reveal significant side-to-side differences.

Pain relief following sesamoidectomy is often incomplete. In the early 1930s, Inge and Ferguson[22] found that only 41% of patients achieved complete pain relief. Mann and colleagues[17,20] reported complete pain relief in 50% of their patients. Brodsky[20] noted 6 of 23 patients had mild to moderate pain following surgery. Despite these conflicting results of pain relief and function, sesamoidectomy still remains the main surgical option in the treatment of recalcitrant plantar hallucal pain.

Tibial Sesamoidectomy

A longitudinal skin incision is performed slightly plantar to a standard medial midline approach to the hallux. The plantar cutaneous nerve is mobilized and protected throughout the procedure. A longitudinal capsulotomy is performed to inspect the articular surface of the metatarsal and sesamoid (**Fig. 10**). This capsulotomy is then repaired and the excision of the sesamoid is performed through an extra-articular approach. The sesamoid is exposed though a plantar incision in line with the fibers of the flexor hallucis brevis. Tagged sutures are placed into the FHB proximally and distally before the sesamoid is excised. The FHL tendon is retracted and protected. After the sesamoid is excised and removed, the defect is repaired to restore the FHB complex. If there is a significant soft tissue defect, an advancement procedure of the abductor hallucis can be performed. The tendon of the abductor hallucis is separated from the medial capsule in a proximally based flap and rotated plantarly to fill the defect of the sesamoidectomy. This can be an effective adjunct to a sesamoidectomy in an athlete with compromised plantar tissues from a chronic "turf-toe."[21]

Postoperative management consists of heel weight bearing for 2 weeks. At the 2-week mark, the patient is allowed to full weight bear in a protective shoe with a toe-spacer or a fracture boot brace. Range of motion is instituted at 4 weeks and at 6 weeks patients are allowed to attempt to wear an accommodative shoe.

Fibular Sesamoidectomy

For advanced deterioration of a fibular sesamoid, sesamoidectomy has been described through either a dorsal or plantar approach. The plantar approach was previously thought to have difficulties with wound healing and painful scar formation.

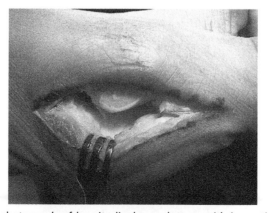

Fig. 10. Operative photograph of longitudinal capsulotomy with inspection of metatarsal-sesamoid articulation.

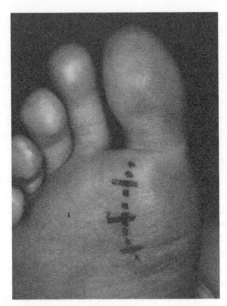

Fig. 11. Plantar incision for fibular sesamoidectomy.

Richardson and colleagues[23] showed a 96% satisfaction rate in 115 patients with 150 plantar incisions for various forefoot procedures. Furthermore, Lin and colleagues[24] demonstrated that the extent and reproducibility of adductor releases through a dorsal approach may be inconsistent and unpredictable, with injury occurring to surrounding structures because of difficulty in visualizing the appropriate anatomic structures. The author's preferred approach is therefore plantar.

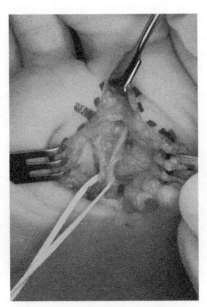

Fig. 12. Plantar approach with nerve isolated and protected.

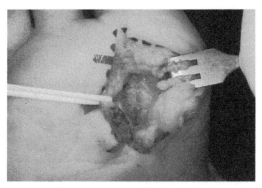

Fig. 13. Plantar defect closed after sesamoid excision.

A plantar incision allows for direct visualization of the sesamoid and surrounding soft tissue structures, minimizes the violation of normal anatomic structures, and provides for repair of the flexor hallucis brevis tendon following sesamoid excision.[25] Also, it should be noted that preserving the adductor mechanism can be difficult through a dorsal approach.

A plantar incision is made along the plantar hallucal crease. Dissection is performed with particular care to protect the flexor hallucis longus tendon and the lateral hallucal branch of the medial plantar sensory nerve (**Figs. 11, 12**). The plantar hallucal nerve is protected throughout the case with gentle retraction using a vessel loop. The sesamoid is circumferentially dissected free with a beaver blade and removed. Meticulous soft tissue repair of the created defect is performed as well as preservation of the adductor hallucis tendon (**Fig. 13**). The skin is approximated with nonabsorbable sutures avoiding subcutaneous nonabsorbable suture material beneath the plantar skin. The foot is placed in a bunion-type bandage/dressing with the hallux held in slight plantar flexion. Postoperatively, the patient is kept non–weight bearing for 2 weeks, and protected for 6 weeks total in a postop walking shoe. Sutures are removed at 2 weeks postoperatively. A custom-molded orthotic device is used as necessary for return to activities.

Milia and colleagues[25] reported on 12 patients treated with fibular sesamoidectomy through a plantar approach. There were no cases of painful scar formation or wound-healing difficulties. A total of 75% of the patients were very satisfied, but the time to recovery can last up to 6 months postoperatively. Three patients suffered from transient parasthesia of the plantar sensory nerve.

SUMMARY

Sesamoid disorders are common pathologic entities involving the first metatarsal phalangeal joint. These clinical disorders range from acute trauma to repetitive injuries that cause stress fractures or avascular necrosis. The hallmark of treatment is initial conservative measures followed by operative treatment if these measures fail. Although the mechanical function of the sesamoids in protecting the plantar structures and providing increased force for great toe plantar flexion is important, resection of the sesamoids can be a very effective treatment option in relieving pain and restoring function. Care must be taken to identify and address any contributing mechanical factors when treating sesamoid disorders to avoid poor outcomes and further mechanical problems such as iatrogenic transfer lesions.

REFERENCES

1. Demond BT, Cory JW, McBryde A. The hallucal sesamoid complex. J Am Acad Orthop Surg 2006;14(13):745–53.
2. Leventen EO. Sesamoid disorders and treatment. Clin Orthop 1991;269:236–40.
3. Richardson EG. Hallucal sesamoid pain: causes and surgical treatment. J Am Acad Orthop Surg 1999;7(4):270–8.
4. Richardson EG. Injuries to the hallucal sesamoids in the athlete. Foot Ankle 1987; 7(4):229–44.
5. Sobel M, Hashimoto J, Arnoczky SP, et al. The microvasculature of the sesamoid complex. Foot Ankle 1992;13(6):359–63.
6. Chamberland PD, Smith JW, Fleming LL. The blood supply to the great toe sesamoids. Foot Ankle 1993;14(8):435–41.
7. Pretterkleiber ML, Wanivenhaus A. The arterial supply of the sesamoid bones of the hallux. Foot Ankle 1992;13(1):27–31.
8. Grace DL. Sesamoid problems. Foot Ankle Clin 2000;5(3):609–27.
9. Potter HG, Pavlov H, Abrahams TG. The hallux sesamoids revisited. Skeletal Radiol 1992;21:437–44.
10. Karasick D, Schweitzer ME. Disorders of the hallux sesamoid complex: MR features. Skeletal Radiol 1998;27:411–8.
11. Biedert R, Hinterman B. Stress fractures of the medial great toe sesamoid in athletes. Foot Ankle Int 2003;24(2):137–41.
12. Blundell CM, Nicholson P, Blackney MW. Percutaneous screw fixation for fractures of the sesamoid bones of the hallux. J Bone Joint Surg Br 2002;84(08):1138–41.
13. McBryde AM Jr, Anderson RB. Sesamoid foot problems in the athlete. Clin Sports Med 1988;7(1):51–60.
14. Scranton PE Jr. Pathologic anatomic variations in the sesamoids. Foot Ankle 1981;1(6):321–6.
15. Aper RL, Saltzman CL, Brown TD. The effect of halux sesamoid resection on the effective moment of the flexor hallucis brevis. Foot Ankle Int 1994;15(9):462–70.
16. Aper RL, Saltzman CL, Brown TD. The effect of halux sesamoid excision on the flexor hallucis longus moment arm. Clin Orthop Relat Res 1996;325:209–17.
17. Mann RA, Coughlin MJ, Baxter D. Sesamoidectomy of the great toe. Orthopaedic Transactions 1985;9:62–3.
18. Coughlin MJ. Surgery of the foot. In: Mann RA, Coughlin MJ, editors. St. Louis (MO): CV Mosby; 1993. p. 494.
19. Mann RA, Coughlin MJ. Hallux valgus—etiology, anatomy, treatment and surgical considerations. Clin Orthop 1981;151:31–41.
20. Brodsky J. Sesamoid excision for chronic non-union, AOFAS Annual Meeting 1991. In: Mann RA, Coughlin MJ, editors. Surgery of the foot. St. Louis (MO): CV Mosby; 1993. p. 498.
21. Lee S, James WC, Cohen BE, et al. Evaluation of hallux alignment and functional outcome after isolated tibial sesamoidectomy. Foot Ankle Int 2005;26(10):803–9.
22. Inge GAL, Ferguson AB. Surgery of the sesamoid bones of the great toe. Arch Surg 1933;27:466–88.
23. Richardson EG, Brotzman SB, Graves SC. The plantar incision for procedures involving the forefoot. J Bone Joint Surg Am 1993;75(5):726–31.
24. Lin I, Bonar SK, Anderson RB, et al. Distal soft tissue release using direct and indirect approaches: an anatomic study. Foot Ankle Int 1996;17(8):458–63.
25. Milia M, Anderson RB, Cohen BE. Plantar approach for fibular sesamoidectomy. Techniques in Foot and Ankle Surgery 2003;2(4):268–71.

Arthroscopy of the Hallux

Dominic S. Carreira, MD

KEYWORDS

• Great toe • Hallux • Metatarsophalangeal • Arthroscopy

Advances in small joint arthroscopes and instrumentation have enabled surgeons to better access and treat various pathologies, while minimizing iatrogenic injury. Many of the techniques employed in small joint arthroscopy have been borrowed from experience in other joints, such as the ankle. As with other joints, interest in arthroscopy of the hallux has increased in recent years. The frequency of arthroscopy of the first metatarsophalangeal (MTP) joint remains limited as compared with other joints. Ferkel reported a rate of 4% (22/541) when accounting for all foot and ankle procedures performed arthroscopically.[1]

First described by Watanabe and colleagues[2] in 1972 in both the MTP and interphalangeal (IP) joints, hallux arthroscopy initially was implemented in the treatment of cartilage lesions. Bartlett[3] noted a single case report of the successful treatment of an osteochondral defect of the metatarsal head in 1982. Ferkel and Van Buecken[4] were the first to present their technique and results on a series of patients in 1991. Similar developments occurred in veterinary medicine, with Yovich and McIlwraith[5] reporting debridement of osteochondral lesions of the comparable joint (fetlock) in horses in 1986.

Proposed advantages of arthroscopic techniques include decreased bleeding, infection rates, and scarring, along with improved cosmesis and quicker recovery and rehabilitation.[6,7] There have been no studies comparing arthroscopic versus open approaches in the first MTP joint specifically.

ANATOMY

An understanding of the gross and arthroscopic anatomy of the hallux is important when considering arthroscopic intervention. The first MTP joint is a chondroid joint composed of the metatarsal head and neck, the proximal phalanx, and the medial and lateral sesamoids. Minimal stability is provided by the articulation because the ball (metatarsal head) and socket (proximal phalanx) are shallow. The sesamoid complex consists of two sesamoid bones, eight ligaments, and seven muscles. The sesamoids are contained within the tendons of the flexor hallucis brevis and articulate

Broward Health Orthopedics, 300 SE 17th St, First Floor, Fort Lauderdale, FL 33316, USA
E-mail address: dcarreira@gmail.com

Foot Ankle Clin N Am 14 (2009) 105–114
doi:10.1016/j.fcl.2008.11.004
1083-7515/08/$ – see front matter © 2009 Elsevier Inc. All rights reserved.

foot.theclinics.com

with the undersurface of the metatarsal head. Both sesamoids are attached on the plantar side through a fibrocartilaginous plate, which allows for smooth gliding. The plantar plate also has attachments to the deep transverse intermetatarsal ligaments, the flexor tendon sheaths, the plantar aponeurosis, and the transverse head of the adductor hallucis. The proper digital nerve lies deep to the transverse metatarsal ligament. The intersesamoid ligament is strong and retains the relationship between the sesamoids. The extensor hallucis longus tendon divides the dorsal joint surface in half, and branches of the deep peroneal nerve innervate the lateral half of the hallux while branches of the superficial peroneal nerve innervate the medial half.

BIOMECHANICS

Active range of motion of the hallux MTP joint in dorsiflexion averages 51° and in plantarflexion 23°. Additional passive range of motion in dorsiflexion averages 23°. In the hallux interphalangeal joint, the active flexion averages 46° and extension to 12°, with additional passive dorsiflexion of 22°.[8] During gait, the maximum joint reaction force noted at the hallux metatarsophalangeal joint is between 40% and 80% body weight.[9] These forces increase significantly with running and jumping, as has been verified by pedobarographic studies.[10] Limitations in motion may be caused by arthritis, impingement by dorsal osteophytes, scar formation after surgery, or after prolonged immobilization following trauma. Altered force distribution may lead to secondary problems, such as lateral forefoot pain, interdigital neuritis, or synovitis as a compensatory mechanism to avoid loading and push off by the hallux.

Physical Examination of the Metatarsophalangeal Joint

A detailed physical examination should be performed to assess for swelling, joint-line tenderness, stiffness, and crepitus. Dorsiflexion and plantarflexion of the MTP and IP joints are checked in the neutral, resting position. Hypermobility of the first ray may be assessed by securing the metatarsal neck between the index finger and thumb, then stabilizing the lateral forefoot with the opposite hand. Instability is detected as increased motion, in the sagittal and/or transverse planes. Pain at end range of motion as compared with throughout mid-range may also be useful in deciding whether osteophyte excision, chondroplasty, or arthrodesis is best indicated.[11]

Indications

Indications for arthroscopy continue to develop. There are no published studies on hallux IP arthroscopy. The published studies on MTP arthroscopy are case reports or small case series [2,11–16] and there are no randomized studies. A number of pathologic conditions have been treated with hallux MTP arthroscopy, the most common of which include: hallux rigidus, focal chondral defects, loose bodies, arthrofibrosis, and synovitis. The few available studies in the literature report favorable outcomes for these indications; these results are discussed in detail later in this chapter. Other less common indications for hallux MTP arthroscopy include: sesamoid pathology, gout, and joint infection. For these pathologies arthroscopic treatment is considered investigational. Contraindications to arthroscopy include: the presence of large osteophytes, severe swelling, arterial insufficiency, soft tissue infection, and soft tissue compromise.

Preoperative Planning

Radiographic examination with standing views of the foot is recommended. These include anteroposterior, lateral, and oblique views. An axial or tangential view of the sesamoids can visualize the metatarsosesamoid articulation. Evaluation of radiographs can identify signs of arthritis, including joint space narrowing and osteophyte formation. MR imaging or CT scanning may be useful in determining the presence of focal osteochondral defects or other associated pathologies. Expectations regarding postoperative level of function should also be explored. In borderline cases in which cheilectomy versus arthrodesis is being considered, an intraoperative decision may be warranted. This option should be discussed preoperatively.

Portal Anatomy

Two portals have been commonly described for hallux MTP arthroscopy. The dorsomedial portal is placed at the joint line just medial to the extensor hallucis longus (EHL) tendon. When placing this portal, care must be taken not to damage the medial dorsal cutaneous branch of the superficial peroneal nerve. The dorsolateral portal is placed at the joint line also, just lateral to the EHL (**Fig. 1**).

Additional portals include the straight medial portal, which is placed halfway between the dorsal and plantar extent of the joint line, and a proximal medial portal, which is placed approximately 4 cm proximal to the MTP joint line between the abductor hallucis tendon and the medial head of the flexor halluxis brevis. This proximal medial portal is more easily established with plantarflexion of the first MTP joint. Lastly, an occasional plantar portal may be established directly centrally.

Diagnostic Arthroscopy

Ferkel has described a 13-point arthroscopic examination of the MTP joint through the dorsolateral portal, which is used to make a systematic evaluation of potential pathologies. This is followed by a 5-point examination through the medial portal to better visualize the posterior plantar capsule, the medial and lateral sesamoids, the central metatarsal head, and the dorsal capsular structures (**Figs. 2 and 3**).

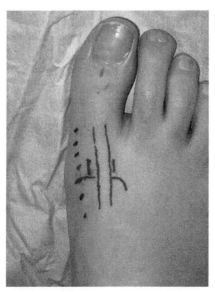

Fig. 1. Dorsomedial and dorsolateral arthroscopic portals of first metatarsophalangeal joint. Dotted line represents dorsomedial cutaneous nerve to the hallux. Extensor hallucis longus (EHL) tendon is central (*longitudinal parallel lines*).

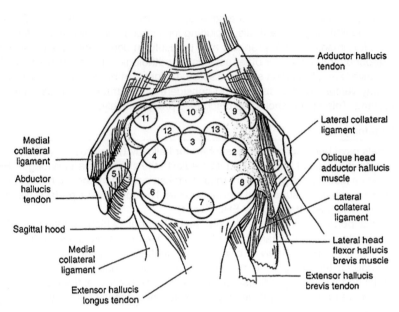

Fig. 2. The 13-point exaqmination of the great toe metatarsal joint viewed through the dorso-lateral portal. (1) lateral gutter; (2) lateral corner of the metatarsal head; (3) central portion of the metatarsal head; (4) medial portion of the metatarsal head; (5) medial gutter; (6) medial capsular reflection; (7) central bare spot; (8) lateral capsular reflection; (9) medial portion of the proximal phalanx; (10) central portion of the proximal phalanx; (11) lateral portion of the central phalanx, (12) medial sesamoid; (13) lateral sesamoid. (*From* Ferkel RD. Arthroscopy of the foot and ankle. In: Coughlin MJ, Mann RA, Saltzman CL, editors. Surgery of the Foot and Ankle, 8th edition. Philadelphia: Mosby Elsevier; 2007; with permission.)

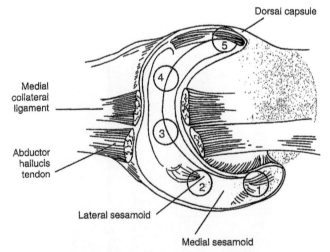

Fig. 3. Great toe metatarsophalangeal joint 5-point examination viewed from the medial portal with the sagittal head removed. (1) posterior plantar capsule; (2) the medial and lateral sesamoids; (3) the central metatarsal head; (4) the superior metatarsal head; (5) the dorsal capsular structures. (*From* Ferkel RD. Arthroscopy of the foot and ankle. In: Coughlin MJ, Mann RA, Saltzman CL, editors. Surgery of the Foot and Ankle, 8th edition. Philadelphia: Mosby Elsevier; 2007; with permission.)

Traction and Instrumentation

Traction may be placed manually through a sterile finger trap device, suspended from an IV holder, or through a pulley system attached to the opposite side of the table (**Fig. 4**). Sufficient weight is used to adequately suspend the lower extremity, typically about 10 lbs. It is helpful to test the size of the finger trap in the clinic before surgery to ensure proper fit. The most useful sizes of arthroscopes include the short 1.9 mm and 2.7 mm, 30- and 70-degree. Care must be taken with these small arthroscopes to prevent breakage. The most useful sizes of the instruments include 2.0-mm and 2.3-mm diameter. Available instrumentation should include shavers, burrs, baskets forceps, graspers, and microfracture awls. In cases where noninvasive distraction is unlikely to be sufficient, it may be necessary to consider open surgery instead.

Surgical Technique

The patient is placed in the supine position and several different types of anesthesia may be administered, including a regional block and general anesthesia. The use of a tourniquet is optional, and may depend on the extent of the procedure. First, the dorsolateral portal is established, because it is the safest portal. With an 18-gauge needle and 3–4 mL of 1% lidocaine or saline solution, the joint is injected to confirm adequate placement. The "nick and spread" technique is used to enter the capsule for each of the portals. An 11 blade is used to incise the skin only, and a mosquito clamp is used to prevent injury to the neurovascular structures and to enter the joint. The jaws of the clamp are then opened to widen the opening in the capsule (**Fig. 5**). The remaining portals are established under direct visualization. A pump system may be used to provide flow and to maintain joint distension. Stabilization of the foot by an assistant is necessary to minimize motion of the foot. A "bump" under each elbow is recommendable for the surgeon to optimize control of fine movements.

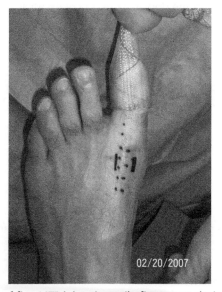

Fig. 4. Manual traction of first MTP joint via sterile finger-trap device.

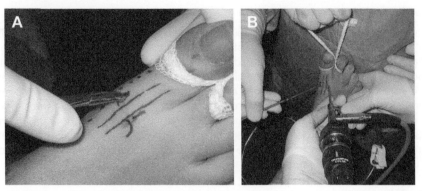

Fig. 5. (*A*) Spreading of subcutaneous tissue and capsule with hemostat. (*B*) Arthroscope in dorsolateral portal with dorsomedial working portal.

DORSAL OSTEOPHYTE EXCISION
Indications and Contraindications

A cheilectomy may be performed arthroscopically for small- to medium-sized dorsal spurs. Contraindications include diffuse degenerative arthritis with joint space loss and extensive periarticular spurring. The precise extent of articular cartilage injury, which precludes arthroscopic treatment, has yet to be determined. Patient age, functional activity levels, and shoewear preferences may factor into the decision making process.

Technique

Inflow can be placed through a medial portal; the arthroscope and instrumentation are placed interchangeably through the dorsomedial and dorsolateral portals. A power shaver is used to remove fibrosis and synovitis (**Fig. 6**). A small elevator is used to elevate the soft tissues off the dorsal spurs, to create additional space for capsular

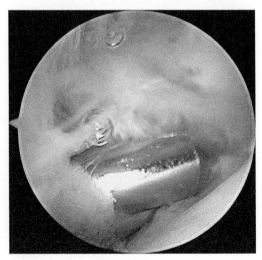

Fig. 6. Arthroscopic synovectomy of first MTP joint.

distension and visualization, and to create a plane of resection. A small, curved-tipped electrocautery with suction is aimed toward the bone and serves to further define this plane of resection while maintaining hemostasis. A 2.0 joint burr then is used to remove bone and the dorsal metatarsal articular surface, with the extent of resection determined in part by improvements in dorsiflexion range of motion. Removal of traction for the dorsal bone resection is useful in that it allows for dorsiflexion of the MTP joint and an increased working space. Intraoperative fluoroscopy may be helpful in guiding the extent of resection.

Technique of Chondroplasty

When treating articular cartilage injuries, a complete diagnostic examination should be performed, and any associated loose bodies should be removed. For focal chondral defects, creation of a stable rim of cartilage can be performed using a shaver and curettes (**Fig. 7**A). Microfracture or drilling techniques, as described for grade IV focal chondral defects in the knee and shoulder,[12,13] also may be applied in the MTP joint (**Fig. 7**B).

Technique of Lysis of Adhesions

A high-angle electrocautery ablation device allows for visualization of the takedown of the scar. The scar removal should be performed in layers so as to avoid over-resection and damage to the adjacent neurovascular structures. The author recommends manipulation under anesthesia following arthroscopic treatment, as doing so before scar removal would create excessive bleeding and creates difficulty with arthroscopic visualization.

Technique of Arthrodesis

To determine the optimal angle for entry and joint preparation, a fluoroscopic image may be obtained. The central plantar portal may be useful for preparation of the plantar aspect of the joint. Along with a freer elevator, a high-angle electrocautery device may be used to identify the margins of the articulation. A 2.9-mm shaver and hooded burr are used to resect soft tissue and bone, with attention to removing all sclerotic areas of opposing bone and to contouring of the arthrodesis site in a cup and cone fashion. Patient debridement of bony and cartilaginous debris is necessary.

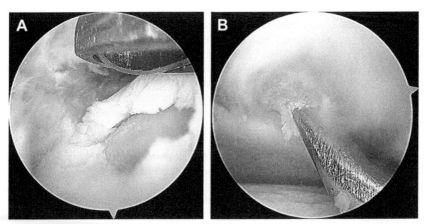

Fig. 7. (A) Creation of stable rim around full-thickness chondral lesion. (B) Microfracture of chondral lesion.

The finger trap distraction is removed, and two 4.0-mm diameter screws are placed percutaneously for fixation.

GUIDELINES FOR POSTOPERATIVE CARE

All wounds are sutured with a nonabsorbable monofilament suture. Options for postoperative footwear include the use of a postoperative shoe with partial weight-bearing or a wedge shoe with full weight-bearing on the heel. The first follow-up visit is scheduled between 7 and 14 days and the sutures are removed. The appropriate timing for the initiation of strengthening and motion is unclear, particularly in the setting of lysis of adhesion or cheilectomy. As long as the wounds are healing well, motion and strengthening may be initiated after the first postoperative visit, although Lui has challenged this approach and described mobilization as early as the first postoperative day.[14] For an MTP arthrodesis, motion and strengthening are initiated approximately 6 weeks following surgery, after there is evidence of bony consolidation. With the exception of an MTP arthrodesis, a stiff-soled shoe may be initiated after pain and swelling have subsided significantly at approximately 4 weeks.

RESULTS

In a series of 22 patients treated with first MTP arthroscopy, Ferkel reported 74% good to excellent, 13% (3) fair, and 13% (3) poor results with a minimum two-year follow-up. Pathologies treated included: degenerative joint disease disease (5), arthrofibrosis (4), synovitis (3), osteophytes (3), osteochondral lesions of the metatarsal head (3), loose bodies (3), and chondromalacia (2). The six patients with fair or poor results all had significant joint degenerative arthritis. Forty-one percent of these patients had prior surgery and there were no complications related to the procedure.[1]

Van Dijk and colleagues published on 25 arthroscopies at an average of two-year follow-up (range, 20 to 32 months) with diagnoses of dorsal impingement syndrome (12), hallux rigidus (5), sesamoiditis (5), osteochondritis dissecans (4), and bacterial arthritis (1). Sixteen patients had a strong reduction or complete relief of pain, and three other patients complained of problems only during sports. Twelve patients regained their preoperative level of sports activity. Subjective results were: six–excellent; eight–good; six–fair; and three–poor. Good to excellent results were reported in eight of 12 patients with dorsal impingement; three of four patients in the osteochondral defect group; two of five in the hallux rigidus group; and three of five in the sesamoid group. Medial sesamoid resection was not advantageous in this study. His technique included use of a 2.7-mm arthroscope.[15]

Davies and Saxby reported their results on 12 arthroscopies of the first MTP joint at a mean follow-up of 19.3 months. The indication for surgery was persistent pain, swelling, and stiffness at the first MTP joint. At follow-up, all patients had no or minimal pain, decreased swelling, and increased range of motion. In three of these patients, a limited arthrotomy also was performed. Their technique employed a 1.9-mm arthroscope.[16]

There is one published case report on the successful outcome of an arthrodesis of the first MTP joint.[17] Internal fixation was placed through a percuatenous approach. The joint was prepared using a 2.0-mm shaver and burr and two 4.0-mm AO cortical screws were placed under fluoroscopic visualization. Successful fusion was confirmed radiographically by 8 weeks. Regarding the use of arthroscopy in first MTP arthrodesis, Davies and Saxby[16] commented "there is no reason why (it) could not be performed in selected patients in the future" and Ferkel[1] stated "arthrodesis appears feasible in certain isolated cases."

In the treatment of hallux rigidus via arthroscopy, Iqbal and Chana[18] reported on a series of 15 patients ages 27 to 60 years with a mean follow-up of 9.4 months. Radiologic examination demonstrated mild to moderate arthritis of the joint with large dorsal osteophytes. Sixty-six percent of patients noted complete pain relief. Range of motion improved from mean preoperative arc of 28.6° to a mean postoperative arc of 69.3°. No complications were reported and patients returned to a level of nonathletic activity at an average of 3.7 weeks.

Debnath and colleagues[19] reported pain-free results in 95% of 25 feet treated with first MTP arthroscopy at a minimum two-year follow-up. The most common indication was early degenerative disease with mid-range pain with or without dorsal osteophyte impingement (12 of 25). Mean preoperative and postoperative American Orthopedic Foot and Ankle Society Hallux MTP and IP scores improved from 43 (range, 10–78) to 97 (range, 87–100). The mean increase in first MTP dorsiflexion was from 8° to 30°. Five of the patients had more definitive procedures after 2 years, including three patients who underwent MTP arthroplasty.

Complications

Reported complications in the literature are limited to neuropraxias, which were reported in two separate studies,[15,19] each of which reported two transient cases. Debnath and colleagues[19] reported recovery within 2 months of the two dorsomedial neuropraxias in their study.

Additional possible procedure-related complications include iatrogenic articular cartilage injury, arthroscope and instrument breakage, infection, wound dehiscence, sinus tract formation, and under- or over-boney resection (in the treatment of hallux rigidus). The use of cannulas to avoid repetitive trauma to the soft tissues on re-entry and limited resection of the soft tissues about the portals may help prevent a number of these complications.

SUMMARY

Arthroscopy of the first MTP joint is a useful, minimally invasive technique in treating a number of pathologies about the hallux MTP joint. However, it is a technically demanding procedure for which there is a learning curve. The small arthroscope and instrumentation are delicate and vulnerable to damage. Practice on cadavers is very useful in shortening this learning curve, and experience with arthroscopy in other joints facilitates the transition to the hallux. In the future, additional studies will help to more specifically define the indications and expected outcomes of treatment as such will help to further elucidate the potential benefits over open surgery.

REFERENCES

1. Ferkel RD. Great toe arthroscopy. In: Whipple TL, editor. Arthroscopy, the foot and ankle. Philadelphia: Lippincott-Raven; 1996. p. 255–72.
2. Watanabe M. Selfox-arthroscope. In: Watanabe No. 24 Arthroscope (Monograph). Tokyo: Teishin Hospital; 1972. p. 46–53.
3. Bartlett DH. Arthroscopic management of osteochondritis disseca. Arthroscopy 1988;4(1):51–4.
4. Ferkel RD, Van Breuken KP. Great toe arthroscopy: indications, technique, and results. Presented at the Arthroscopy Association of North America, San Diego, 1991.

5. Yovich JV, McIlwraith CW. Arthroscopic surgery for osteochondral fractures of the proximal phalanx, the metacarpal-phalangeal and metatarsophalangeal joint in horses. J Am Vet Med Assoc 1986;188:273.

6. Morgan CD, Cascells CD. Arthroscopic-assisted glenohumeral arthrodesis. Arthroscopy 1992;8:262–6.

7. Myerson MS, Quill G. Ankle arthrodesis: a comparison of an arthroscopic and an open method of treatment. Clin Orthop 1991;268:84–95.

8. Myerson M, Shereff M. The pathological anatomy of claw and hammer toes. J Bone Joint Surg Am 1989;71:45–9.

9. Hutton WC, Dhanendran M. The mechanics of normal and hallux valgus feet a quantitative study. Clin Orth Relat Res 1981;157:7–13.

10. Salzman C, Nawoczenski D. Complexities of foot architecture as a base of support. Foot Ankle Ther Res 1995;21:354–60.

11. Coughlin MJ, Shurnas PS. Hallux rigidus. J Bone Joint Surg Am. 2004;86(Suppl 1 Pt 2):119–30.

12. Steadman J, Briggs K, Rodrigo J, et al. Outcomes of microfracture in traumatic chondral defects of the knee: average 11-year followup. Arthroscopy 2003;19: 477–84.

13. Huffard BH, Horan MP, Millet PJ, et al. Outcomes of full-thickness articular cartilage injuries of the shoulder treated with microfracture. Arthroscopy 2007; 23(Suppl):24–5.

14. Lui TH. Arthroscopic release of first metatarsophalangeal arthrofibrosis. Arthroscopy 2004;22(8):901–6.

15. Dijk van CN, Veenstra KM, Nuesch BC. Arthroscopic surgery of the metatarsophalangeal first joint. Arthroscopy 1998;14:851–5.

16. Davies MS, Saxby TS. Arthroscopy of the first metatarsophalangeal joint. J Bone Joint Surg Br 1999;81(2):203–6.

17. Carro LP, Vallina BB. Arthroscopic-assisted first metatarsophalangeal joint arthrodesis. Arthroscopy 1999;15(2):215–7.

18. Iqbal MJ, Chana GS. Arthroscopic cheiliectomy for hallux rigidus. Arthroscopy 1998;14(3):307–10.

19. Debnath UK, Hemmady MV, Hariharan K. Indications for and technique of first MTP arthroscopy. Foot Ankle Int 2006;27(12):1049–54.

Index

Note: Page numbers of article titles are in **boldface** type.

A

foot.theclinics.com

Moving?

Make sure your subscription moves with you!

To notify us of your new address, find your **Clinics Account Number** (located on your mailing label above your name), and contact customer service at:

E-mail: elspcs@elsevier.com

800-654-2452 (subscribers in the U.S. & Canada)
314-453-7041 (subscribers outside of the U.S. & Canada)

Fax number: 314-523-5170

Elsevier Periodicals Customer Service
11830 Westline Industrial Drive
St. Louis, MO 63146

*To ensure uninterrupted delivery of your subscription, please notify us at least 4 weeks in advance of move.

Printed and bound by CPI Group (UK) Ltd, Croydon, CR0 4YY

03/10/2024

01040452-0017